Autophagy for Beginners

The Amazing Anti-Aging Secrets of Combining Intermittent Fasting & The Keto Diet

I0135619

Written By

Jason Michaels

&

Thomas Hawthorn

© Copyright 2019 - All rights reserved.

Medical Disclaimer

This book is not intended as a substitute for the medical advice of physicians. The reader should regularly consult a physician in matters relating to his/her health and particularly with respect to any symptoms that may require diagnosis or medical attention.

Please consult your physician before starting any diet or exercise program.

Any recommendations given in this book are not a substitute for medical advice.

Contents

Ketogenic Autophagy

Combine the Keto Diet & Nobel Prize Winning Science to Look and Feel Younger, Lose Weight and Extend Your Life + 28 Day OMAD Meal Plan

Written By

Thomas Hawthorn

Introduction

Think of the most popular pairs in history.

Carrot and peas. Salt and pepper. Captain America and Iron Man (or Thor and Hulk for you Asgardian fans). Tom and Hardy. Charlize and Theron.

They go so well together.

And that is exactly what happens when you put autophagy with ketogenesis, they go well together. They complement each other. I do not mean that in a metaphysical or philosophical way. There is a scientific foundation for my conclusions about autophagy and ketogenesis.

But what do the aforementioned terms even mean? I am guessing that to some of you, I might as well have introduced them in Japanese because they are not going to make sense without an explanation.

Well, we are going to explore both autophagy and ketogenesis in depth in a later chapter. For now, what you need to understand is that autophagy helps with the consumption of damaged and dangerous cells. In numerous cases, these cells have the potential to turn cancerous. On the other hand, ketogenesis is the process of creating ketone bodies. These help in distributing energy throughout the body.

How are they related?

In a recent study conducted by Japanese scientists on mice, they discovered that when they removed the gene that causes autophagy from the rodents, their ketone levels dropped as well.

Author, you say.

Those are mice, you say. How can they be of significance to us?

There is a reason why laboratories utilize mice in medical testing; they share genetic and biological traits that are close to human beings. It is for this reason that many medicines are first tested out on mice before moving on to human trials.

So far, we do not have any studies about autophagy with ketogenesis performed on humans. Nevertheless, there is an interesting conclusion that one can draw here that intermittent fasting helps with autophagy, which in turn contributes to ketogenesis in the body.

Now you are wondering about the fact that we haven't yet established the connection between fasting and autophagy.

We don't have to.

The US National Library of Medicine National Institutes of Health has done the legwork for us.

According to the world's largest medical library, the ritual of having three meals a day (with a little snacking added in by some people) is not a natural habit and does not provide the human body any benefits. This is because our ancestors – the hunters and the gatherers – did not have the luxury of eating so frequently during the day.

Which is why their bodies would go through a fasting period several times during the day. The body, under the stress of fasting, would, of course, try to protect itself. It did this by removing any cells that could potentially cause the body harm due to the lack of food. This eventually led to the destruction of numerous dangerous cells throughout the body. In short, our ancestors – without having realized it – forced their bodies to cleanse themselves.

In today's world, we are fixated on getting our daily fix of food. This is probably because of the fact that we were taught to have breakfast, lunch, and dinner to stave off hunger. And the practice worked! After all, who likes to stay hungry?

As we grew up, we never really questioned the whole idea of eating so regularly during the day. It never occurred to us that there is a way to have a proper diet that could benefit us and our bodies.

After all, our parents and practically society itself had convinced us to adopt a habit that we never questioned. That is not a bad thing at all. They were concerned about our health and they might not have been aware of autophagy.

However, science has made significant progress during the years. And we can easily become aware of numerous ideas, facts, and studies regarding our health, body, and well-being at the click of a button and a few keystrokes.

Take for example the 2016 Nobel Prize-winning study conducted by Yoshinori Ohsumi, a Japanese cell biologist. He discovered that during fasting, the cells break down various proteins and other materials in our body and turn them into energy. Furthermore, the cells also eliminate invading bacteria and viruses and send them off for recycling. This process of the cell turning materials into energy and recycling harmful components in our body is known as autophagy.

Not many people know about this process, even though it is renowned in the medical community (it won the Nobel Prize after all).

However, if people were made aware of autophagy, then we would have many who would understand just how important intermittent fasting is.

Additionally, when you combine fasting with the ketogenic diet, you are giving the body not only the chance to remove harmful materials but to intake the right materials as well.

See what I mean about how the two processes of autophagy and ketogenesis are an incredible pair?

That is what we shall be focusing on in this book.

I am not here to take you down a confusing labyrinth of complex medical terms and studies. I am here to show you just how important intermittent fasting is for a wholesome life. I am here to give you tips on how you can adopt this method of fasting into your life, how you do not have to give up on your workout regime or fitness routines for the purpose of fasting, and how you can change your life for the better.

I will also guide you through the OMAD, or One Meal a Day, process. You will even learn about why traditional dieting techniques are not exactly benefiting you in any way.

You will become aware of a powerful tool to enable you to unlock the healing potential of your body.

You hold in your hands a compendium that will change the way you see dieting and personal well-being.

On that note, I bid you welcome to the world of Ketogenic Autophagy.

Think of the process as a keto diet on steroids, but instead of causing harm, it is going to cleanse your body.

Chapter 1: Why the Traditional North American Diet is Killing You

You know that when a study involving the eating habits of an entire country becomes newsworthy, then you should probably take notice. Especially if you are residing within said country.

The study we are talking about was conducted by the Journal of the American Medical Association. It garnered so much attention that Time, CBS News, Yahoo!, and even U.S. News covered the topic.

To give to a bit of background and show you the level of seriousness of the study, you need to understand that the results took deep insights from earlier research conducted by the U.S. government for a national health survey. It was no surprise that the survey revealed that most people did not consume the recommended amounts of healthy food.

This led to the Journal of the American Medical Association discovering that what is killing most Americans are their bad eating habits. In fact, the study showed that Americans eat too much bacon, consume too much sugar, and eat too few nuts, vegetables, and fruits. This habit of consuming fatty and sugary foods is truly harmful, leading to heart conditions, diabetes, and even weight gain.

That's right, even sugar can cause weight gain.

How, you ask?

Let us start with why food is important.

Your body depends on food for energy.

We all know that.

But apart from that, the body takes proteins from foods to help the cells in your body do their job. Your body requires the fats from foods to produce new cells and hormones, and help with the movement of vitamins. You are going to need the vitamins from foods if you intend to keep your skin healthy and your bones strong.

In many ways, foods affect many different processes in your body. You need water not just because it makes up to anywhere from 50% to up to 66% of your body weight, but because your body uses it to regulate temperature.

In the same way, foods also affect your weight in more ways than you can imagine.

Take the hormone insulin for example. This hormone is responsible for allowing glucose to enter your cells. Whether you have a healthy dose of insulin or you are taking insulin treatment to regulate the levels of the hormone, the result is the same, insulin sends glucose to your cells and this lowers the amount of glucose in your blood.

The calories that you consume provide the glucose that you require and this is where excess sugar becomes a problem.

If you consume more calories or sugar than required, insulin does not transfer the glucose to your cells. They are simply converted to fats.

The result? Weight gain.

People who suffer from diabetes are at the highest risk of this process. Which is why their doctor or dietician recommends them to provide their body with the right nutrients and minimize the amount of sugar they consume.

But that does not mean non-diabetic people cannot suffer the consequences of a poor diet. In fact, they most probably will.

When we think of a rich or healthy diet, we think of adapting something to fit the typical three-meals-a-day scheme. We are so used to the scheme that we cannot imagine parting with it. In fact, we may have all heard the popular quote "breakfast is the most important meal of the day."

It does sound like it makes sense. In fact, it should be right. Right?

Hardly.

Let me start off by saying that the Romans had it correct.

And no, I am not talking about their politics or economics. I am talking about their meal plan.

Indeed. The Romans had a healthy meal plan, though I am not certain if they had a concept of meal plans back in the day. Let us just say that they had proper eating habits.

Confused? Don't be. It will all make sense in a bit.

First, a bit of background before we revert to the Romans.

The idea of breakfast began with cereal. Before the invention of cereal, people did not consume breakfast as frequently and did not make it part of their routine as they do in the present time.

In fact, during the medieval period, only royalties and people of wealth could enjoy breakfast. It was a luxury back then. Common people could not afford to have meals multiple times during the day. Even having two meals was a treat to those who could not afford them (which practically meant a lot of people).

As time moved on, cities began to develop more and more. Technology brought in convenience and an industrial revolution. Life became much busier. Those employees, workers, and professionals who worked according to a schedule did not receive time to have a decent meal during the day.

Their solution? Might as well have something before heading off to work. That way, they would not be too hungry.

And lo and behold, we have breakfast getting more common.

Soon, the concept of breakfast spread to different sections of society. This, in turn, gave rise to a whole new market dedicated to serving a new lifestyle of people having meals in the morning.

Eventually, manufacturers realized that people choose foods that they could quickly eat in the morning without having to cook it. Their answer to that? Cereals.

Fun fact: John Harvey Kellogg was one of the people who spearheaded the cereals movement. However, Kellogg's motivations were a bit, unorthodox, to say the least. You see, he believed that cereals could improve the health of people and stop them from desiring masturbation and sex too much. Thankfully, none of his beliefs made it into the marketing campaign or we would be looking at cereals in a completely different light.

So back to cereals.

No, I am not going to say that they actually do play a role in stopping you from enjoying your, well, "me time".

What I will say is that manufacturers needed a hook to sell the cereals. They needed a strong marketing campaign. They focused on convincing people that breakfast is an essential component of your everyday life. They knew that rather than trying to market the product, they could market the idea itself.

It worked. Eventually, this campaign led to numerous messages on the importance of breakfast. You could see stores handing out pamphlets and radio stations proclaiming, "Nutrition experts believe that breakfast is the most essential meal of the day."

The reality, however, is that scientists haven't been able to land on a conclusive answer. Yes, breakfast does help stave off starvation as in many cases, people have not eaten for quite a while (the time difference between lunch and dinner is marginal). However, the idea that breakfast carries most of the burden of keeping you healthy is not the right one.

The breakfast trend created a whole new market that manufacturers took advantage of. In similar ways, the food industry is always keeping an eye out for lifestyle choices and trends that they can use to generate profit.

Over the decades, new food fads keep on rising. As they accumulate, they lead to what we have today: a complex system of food trends where nobody questions the veracity of the facts that they are being bombarded with. Unlike other countries that have relied on agriculture for generations, Americans do not have the support of earlier generations who have lived on growing food for years. This leads to the development of certain ideas about food that may not be grounded on scientific evidence. In fact, new food fads are cropping up even more in the present and people are confused – and in many cases – misled by the information they receive.

New fads arise because they are based on the complex food habits of Americans. These habits are themselves based on the type of foods commonly consumed by the general masses.

And at the base of the food chain (no pun intended) is corn.

Think that is hard to believe?

Let us take some examples of popular foods consumed by Americans.

Gatorade. Hamburgers. Cheetos.

All of these foods are made using compounds created by corn.

In fact, let us take each of the foods listed above and examine how corn influences them.

Gatorade uses corn syrup. Guess what the major content of that ingredient is.

The American cattle industry uses corn heavily. This is because when animals are fed corn, they take less time to fatten. They are, in turn, used as ingredients for some of the most popular foods out there. Chicken patties. Hamburgers. In fact, think of all the fast food giants like McDonald's, KFC, and Arby's. They need to churn out their products as fast as possible because of the growing demand for their food. To deliver the right amount of supply, they need ingredients such as meat as quickly as possible. This, in turn, encourages industries to use methods to increase the production of meat.

At this point, I don't have to tell you what one of those methods is.

That's right, corn feeding.

What about Cheetos, you ask? Well, some of your favorite snacks are made using enriched corn meal including, you guessed it, Cheetos.

The above three examples that I have provided are just some of the various foods that use corn or a compound of corn.

You might just be thinking, is that all there is to it author? Is that why you are particular about corn?

Far from the truth. In fact, here are a few things you should know about corn in America.

According to SmartMoney, you can find corn in 3 out of every 4 products in the supermarket. Surprised? There is more.

According to data compiled by the U.S. Department of Agriculture, corn is also used by biotech companies. At this point, if you are thinking that perhaps they only consume a little, then think again because the products that use corn as the main input were worth over $125 billion in 2012. Just to give you a sense of scale, the GDP of the country of Angola is predicted by the International Monetary Fund to be around $110 billion in 2019. Think about it, the biotech industry is just one of the many industries that utilize corn. Imagine if we start to combine every industry dependent on corn. This goes to show just how much industries depend on the cereal grain.

According to the National Corn Growers Association, Americans consume more than one-third of all the corn produced in the world. This fact can be combined with another study which has shown that many Americans can attribute over 50 percent of their biomass to corn!

Why am I stating these facts? For one, when so many people depend on corn to such a high degree, then there are definitely going to be brands, companies, and manufacturers ready to meet their demands through various corn-based products. For another, no matter how many facts we present to the world, we might find ourselves facing the growing number of products on the supermarket shelf to show that we might not be getting anywhere with our fact-checks. In fact, when industries realize that science might hamper their profit line, they hire lobbyists to ensure that their production is not threatened. They create a type of "carb craze" to keep people going after their products time and time again. You might not even be aware that this phenomenon of "carb craze" is taking place. When you only see the end results – which are the numerous products available in the market – that are available in your local store or supermarket, it can be difficult to imagine that most of those products are fueled by corn. But that alone is what fuels Americans' dependency on these high carb content products.

Of course, no one would ever manufacture their products under the title of "high" carbs".

I am not sure if people would run after their products if they did something like that.

Nowadays, manufacturers have another food fad or trend that they are after. In fact, you might have seen many products with a special label – low carbs.

That label makes everything sound healthy. People who are looking to reduce their carb consumption are probably thinking what a great alternative low-carb foods can make.

However, those labels are just what they are and nothing more; they are merely labels. You see, if you buy a product that has the label "low carb", there is no assurance that it has a much lower carbohydrate content than other products or foods that do not have such a label. Why is that? Because there are no nutrition cataloging guidelines or legal classifications for low-carbohydrate foods. This means that is it entirely up to the manufacturer to decide what exactly they think low-carb means. And the best part? Low-carb foods are more expensive!

Here is an example: when you purchase a low-carb beer, you are going to consume about 2.6 grams of carbohydrates. When you perform a rough calculation, the whole content of the beer equals 95 calories. If you choose a regular light beer, you are going to consume about 3.2 grams of carbohydrates. That amounts to about 96 calories. For such a dismal amount of difference, you are paying almost 50% to 75% more than your average light beer.

When a new food trend appears, you have an entire industry pouncing upon it to make the most use of it. They want you to purchase their products. They definitely do not want you to adopt a keto diet. Why would they? If you practiced eating healthy food and combine it with intermittent fasting, then who is going to consume all the variety of carb-filled (or so-called "low carb") foods stacked one above the other on your local supermarket shelf?

Over the years, manufacturers have adopted various techniques to sell their products and defend their stance against the growing concern about the ingredients they utilize. Apart from the aforementioned low-carb labels that they attach to their products, they have also gone on to spread information about the harmful effects of proteins. The popular theory is that proteins cause the load of acid in your body to increase. This, in turn, compels the body to take in calcium from your bones to neutralize the acidity levels. The increase in calcium causes problems in your kidneys, a notable example is the formation of kidney stones.

In reality, long-term studies have disproved this idea.

These studies have found that protein intake does not harm the bones and definitely does not damage the kidneys. The opposite is true. Proteins have been known to improve bone density! Let us also not forget the fact that proteins are the building blocks of life! How else do you imagine your cells functioning if they do not have the support of proteins?

You have the power to make informed decisions about your life. You have to understand what information is true and what is just manufactured to make sure you do not change your bad habits.

We just saw how bad habits are affecting the health of an entire nation. We also saw how habits are formed and how manufacturers make use of those habits (also called food fads or trends in the modern jargon) to sell you items that you probably do not need in your life.

Which is why we have a keto diet as your savior.

Chapter 2: Ketosis Without the BS

Let's get the obvious out of the way:

A keto diet is a low-carb and high-fat diet.

You use this diet to make sure that your body burns fat more effectively.

More than 50 studies have been conducted on the diet and results show that the diet benefits a plethora of areas: weight loss, better health, improved physical performance, and more.

Now that is out of the way, let us look at some of the things you might not be aware of about a keto diet. More importantly, what exactly is happening to your body on a daily basis? Sure, you are getting healthier, but shouldn't there be more details?

There are.

When you are on a keto diet, you tend to feel less hungry. Eventually, your body starts producing ketones. Ketones, in turn, assist your body in controlling hormones that affect your appetite. They control the influence of hormones like ghrelin, which is your "hunger" hormone. While doing so, they also enhance the production of cholecystokinin, which is the hormone that gives you the feeling of being "full" or less hungry.

When you combine keto diet's effects on the above hormones, you have a wonderful result. You do not feel like snacking regularly. When we are hungry, we tend to consume whatever we get our hands on. In our minds, we feel that we are merely snacking a small amount to manage our hunger. However, when you add up the little snacks you have been consuming over a period of time such as a month, then you might just notice an alarming result: you have consumed a whopping amount of snacks in total!

A keto diet controls your habit of grabbing small bites regularly, making it easier for you to go longer without food.

Your body then has to reach out to other sources for its energy. Enter your fat reserves. When your body starts consuming your fat, you start losing weight fairly quickly.

But hold on just a minute. Didn't we just say that we are going to focus on a high-fat diet in keto? So are we losing weight just to gain it back?

That is not true.

First of all, let us get something out of the way. Fats are not bad. Your body needs fats. The problem occurs when you consume too much of them.

In a keto diet, you are consuming the right amount of good fats at a specific time in the day, avoiding three-meal a day schemes and unnecessary snacking.

You consume plenty of good fats on a keto diet. This fat helps you remain satiated, preventing you from feeling hunger quickly. Fat also stabilizes your blood sugar levels and prevents you from experiencing extreme fluctuations in your energy levels.

When your body functions by using ketones as a source of fuel, then it has a stable energy source. On the other hand, when your body uses carbs it requires frequent doses of carbs to keep it functioning normally.

Think of the times that you eat a big pack of chips to stave of hunger. You might have eaten the entire pack by yourself but you still find yourself hungry a couple of hours later. Sometimes even sooner. When some people experience this form of hunger, they brush it off thinking that they probably consumed a small number of chips. Far from it. It is not the number of chips that caused the hunger. It is the body's growing dependence on carbs.

When you transition from these carb-filled foods to a keto diet with useful fats, you can power through the day without feeling the need to stare at your refrigerator the way a hungry hyena stares at its new prey.

But to reap the benefits of a keto diet, you cannot expect changes to occur overnight. There is a process that takes place.

Keto-adaption is a multifaceted process. Your body is shifting from the use of glucose, as it has been doing for years, to primarily utilizing ketones and the fat it stores for energy. Your body needs time to accommodate that change. Your body might require longer than a few days to get used to the process.

If you look at the changes occurring on a day-to-day basis, then here is what happens. After two to four days, the blood ketone levels in your body might increase to anywhere from 1 to 2 millimolar, or mM. A millimolar is a measurement used to show how concentrated something is in a solution. During this phase, it might be rather difficult for people to maintain keto's low-carb diet.

Sometimes, it might be more challenging for certain people to adapt to a keto diet. In such cases, they might have to reduce their carb intake even further.

At this point, you might wonder if you can simply make use of any low carb diet. Does that not equate to entering into a state of ketosis?

The reality is far more complex than that.

First, let us seek to understand the difference between a keto diet and a low-carb diet by examining each one independently.

Understanding the Keto Diet

In a ketogenic diet, you are pushing your body to use as few carbs as it can. In many ways, people split their diet into a ratio that shows the percentage of fat, protein, and carbs they consume in a particular day. Generally, the division of nutrients happens in the below percentage:

- Fat: 65% to 80%

- Protein: 15% to 25%

- Carbs: 5% to 10%

Yikes. You might not have been expecting your carb levels to drop that low. But welcome to the keto diet and quite frankly, every part of the diet is necessary. And no, there is no wiggle room for change. You are not going to get an 11% carb rate or a 12% carb rate. However, do note that the ratio of carbohydrates may vary depending on the situation or the diet.

For most people, adopting a keto diet means having below 50 grams of carbs per day. By drastically reducing your intake of carbs, you coax your body into a state of ketosis which then becomes the process that provides the main source of fuel for your body.

Essentially, the percentage split in the diet that I had mentioned earlier meant that:

- You are going to have mostly fat until you are satisfied.

- You are going to get your protein intake because it is essential (do not pay heed to the rumor mill about its harmful effects).

- You are also going to get a small number of calories from carbohydrates.

Through the process of ketosis, you are entering into a unique metabolic state that acts as a response to an energy crisis. The only difference is that you are going to respond to that crisis by ensuring that you have the right materials to supply. Basically, you are changing the selection of fuel for your body. You are taking away something that is not good for you and adding something that benefits you greatly.

Understanding the Low-Carb Diet

One of the primary differences that you can make out between a keto diet and a low-carb diet is that in a low-carb diet, there are no strict levels of carbs you should consume in a day. The idea is to reduce the intake of carbs but there is no specific limit.

Low-carb diets are typically not so low that they push your body in a state of full ketosis. You might enter a mild form of ketosis between your low-carb meals. But remember, that state of mild ketosis only lasts until your next meal. You are going to exit the state real quick. For the most part, you won't enter a full-ketosis mode on a low-carb diet. However, there are certain exceptions to this rule. When you are sleeping, perform a fast, or workout, to highlight a few examples, you might enter into a more intense state of ketosis. However, do note that you more than likely won't be taking advantage of the ketosis process through a low-carb diet. This is because when you enter a specific state and exit it quickly you are not taking advantage of the process. You have to enter ketosis and make sure that you maintain that state for a long period of time and as frequently as possible.

That does not mean that there are no easy techniques or steps you can take to achieve full ketosis. Here are the main tips that you need to be aware of to enter into a state of ketosis:

- The most important part is to minimize your carb intake as much as possible. Remember the 5% to 10% split? That should be your starting point. You could start off at 10% carbs and then reduce as you see fit.

- Try to include coconut oil in your diet. This is because it contains certain fats called medium-chain triglycerides (MCTs). What is different about this fat? Well, MCTs can be easily used by the liver. Once they enter the liver, they can be used as a source of energy or can be turned to ketones. Here is an interesting fact about coconut oil. Research has also shown that consuming coconut oil can be one of the best methods to increase the level of ketones for Alzheimer's disease patients. People with nervous system disorders can also make use of coconut oil to improve ketone levels.

- Increase your physical activity. There are two main reasons for this. One is that ketosis helps you perform better in numerous physical activities, including endurance based sports. The other reason is that physical activities, in turn, help you enter ketosis. It is a wonderful balance and helps you make the most of your diet.

- I mentioned good fats before. You should be focusing on taking in more of such fats. You will need them as a source of energy after all.

- Maintain a proper level of protein intake. Do not consume too much of it. Now, you might think to yourself that what the big companies have been saying was true all along, protein is not good for you. That is not the reason I asked you to maintain your protein intake. Too much of anything is bad for you. Too many carbs? Bad for you. Too much sugar? Definitely not recommended. Too much calcium? You are going to feel the effects of that. In a similar manner, you need to control your protein intake as well. However, the fact still remains that protein is vital for your body.

With all of this mention of keto and low-carb diets, you may wonder how you are going to know if you are actually in a state of ketosis or if you are simply in the process of being on just another diet.

Is there a test to determine the level of ketosis?

As a matter of fact, there is.

If you have heard of the procedure where people utilize strips to take a ketosis test, let me tell you that you won't have to do the same.

Here are a few tell-tale signs:

Breath

When you begin your keto journey, you might experience what people commonly call "keto breath". When your body begins to produce ketone bodies, one of the byproducts of the process is acetone. The smell of this byproduct is rather unique. Some people claim to smell "nail polish" while others claim it has a distinct "fruity" or "metallic" smell to it.

Whatever scent you get from acetone, it stays for just the first few weeks and then disappears after that. You can minimize its effect by brushing or flossing, but you probably won't be able to remove the smell completely.

Weight Loss

Your weight loss might not come as a surprise to you. After all, losing any extra weight is something that we would like to achieve as well. You can experience a fast drop in weight within the first week itself. Many people falsely believe that this happens due to the loss of fat, the reality is that it is the result of the body using up the stored carbs and water.

After the initial drop in your weight, you should notice a continual decrease in your body fat as long as you maintain a state of deficiency in your calorie intake.

Decreased Hunger

Once you are well into a ketogenic diet, you might experience a reduction in your hunger levels. This is a good reaction to the diet. When you do not feel hungry too often, you are not compelled to start thinking about getting a small snack. Though the research behind your decreased hunger is sparse, scientists are still trying to figure out just what causes a keto diet to help you prevent feeling the urge to nibble on some goodies frequently.

Increased Energy

When people adopt a low-carb diet (and not a keto diet), they often report feeling tired and sick easily. However, people who take up a keto diet have noticed increased levels of focus and energy. Do note that it does take a while for you to get used to the diet and notice its effects.

Short-Term Fatigue

When you switch to a keto diet, the initial phase (which comprises the first few weeks), might be the most challenging for people. One of the effects that many people feel is fatigue and weakness.

People who go through such effects often feel like they would prefer quitting the diet altogether. In many cases, people do indeed give up on the diet.

But here is something you should know about the keto diet: fatigue in the beginning is completely normal. Your body has spent decades getting used to one particular diet filled with carbohydrates and now it has to make a switch to another diet devoid of the regular supply of carbs. It is similar to writing using one hand for half your life and then trying to write with the other hand, hoping to master the process in just a single day. It is not going to happen. You need time to get over the initial discomfort before you can make any progress.

The same train of thought applies to a keto diet as well. You might feel discomfort initially, but do not give up on your new food habits. Go along with it for a few weeks and allow your body to acclimatize itself to the new shift in your eating habits.

After all, the end result is worth the change.

Chapter 3: The Relationship Between Ketosis and Autophagy

Did you know that in Greek, the word autophagy actually means to eat one's self?

That sounds rather barbaric, doesn't it? One might think that anything associated with that word is dastardly.

However, there is some truth to the Greek meaning of the word when you use it to describe the process occurring within the body.

When there are no external supplies of food, the body begins to eat itself. However, it does not do this in a horrific way. What actually happens is that your body targets damaged proteins and cells. By destroying these components, the process gives way for newer and healthier cells and proteins to arise in their place.

You are encouraging your body to regenerate.

Doesn't the body always get rid of damaged cells?

It does.

But as we age, we experience stress, more physical activities, burnouts, and other constant pressures of everyday life. This increases the rate at which the cells in our bodies begin to deteriorate. Add the fact that we are feeding our body unhealthy components, and we are not giving it enough of a break to take care of the damaged cells.

This is why autophagy is important: It helps to remove the increasing number of damaged cells from the body, including certain types of cells called senescent cells that have no actual purpose other than lingering inside organs and tissues. One of the main reasons to ensure that we remove damaged and senescent cells from our body is because these cells can activate inflammatory pathways and could become vital factors in the formation of various diseases.

We are better off without them.

Autophagy is not just a weapon against bad cells. You can use it to obtain a lot of advantages for your body. Here are just a few of them.

Bodily Function and Quality of Life

You might have heard the term "anti-aging" being thrown around a lot. It does have its charms and many products claim to provide you with the ability to turn back the clock on your body. Well, that is not entirely possible. However, autophagy has a way to make a type of anti-aging process occur within your body. How does it happen? Since the early 1950s, scientists have been aware of the process of autophagy but it was only recently that they were able to uncover more information about how it improves the health of your cells by replacing the damaged ones, as we had seen before. This process results in the following:

Newer cells mean healthier cells. This means your bodily functions improve tremendously.

When your cells are repaired or replaced, they function much better. This, in turn, means that they behave like newer and younger cells. When they do, you feel and look younger.

Increased Longevity

The above point directly links to another benefit that autophagy provides the body: longevity. When you are replacing damaged cells with healthier (and younger) ones, then you are preventing older cells from taking over your body. When you have old cells, they not only function slowly but they also cause your body to slack and age slightly faster. Think of the times you have seen many people say that they are in their 40s or 50s and you are taken aback simply because they do not look their age. The reason for their youthful appearance and vigor is no miracle product or treatment. It is simply the body getting rid of older proteins and cells. Is autophagy similar to the fountain of youth? Nothing so dramatic I'm afraid. But autophagy does come pretty close to making you feel and look young, minus any invasive procedures.

Reducing Chronic Inflammation

Autophagy helps your body manage its level of inflammation by either boosting or suppressing the degree of immune response that you might require for a given situation. For the most part, autophagy reduces the inflammation caused by your immune response by managing the proteins called antigens that give the signals that activate such responses.

Preventing and Delaying Neurodegenerative Diseases

According to the US National Library of Medicine National Institutes of Health, many neurodegenerative diseases are caused by damaged, or what scientists call "misfolded", proteins. As we have seen how autophagy gets rid of these damaged proteins, the process eventually reduces the severity of various neurodegenerative diseases such as Alzheimer's disease. In many cases, autophagy has also been known to prevent the spread of such diseases across the brain.

Autophagy is our body's superpower. It is the way we can improve our vitality while staving off diseases and health complications. But where does ketosis fit into all of this? How does intermittent fasting lead to better autophagy? Why have celebrities such as Beyonce and Hugh Jackman all gone public about the benefits of keto dieting?

Let us take it from the top once again.

We have already established how fasting helps your body enter a state of ketosis. This way, you are avoiding the dependency on carbs and instead relying on the useful fats that you consume during the fasting period. The process of using useful fat helps your body release chemicals called ketones. The ketones have an important role to play in your brain, where they release an essential protein called Brain-derived neurotrophic factor, or BDNF. One of the many purposes of BDNF is to build and reinforce neurons and neural pathways in those areas of the brain that are focused on memory and learning. This is probably why a lot of people claim to have a better capacity to retain information and an improved learning process when they enter a keto diet.

So far, so good. We have fasting based on a keto diet releasing all the good stuff in your body.

We have also seen how fasting triggers autophagy and gets rid of the harmful proteins and cells in your body. But when you add ketosis to the equation, then what really happens is that you remove your body's dependency on carbs. You see, carbs actually delay the autophagy process by days because they are your body's primary source of fuel. They cannot be recycled quickly enough.

Ketosis, on the other hand, increases the use of fats. This, in turn, makes the body less dependent on carbs. Which means you do not feel compelled to eat as often as you used to. And when you can manage your eating habits, your body is ready to enter the autophagy phase. You are then ready to eat less and live better.

And that is how the magic happens.

Nevertheless, we often look at calories like a criminal that needs to be given a life sentence. They are not completely bad. In fact, if you are aiming to lose weight, then you have to make note of something important: calories are units of energy. When you take the factor of energy into consideration, then you should realize your body does need energy. It just needs a calorie deficit diet to provide with enough energy to keep you going while you use up the energy in your fat stores. You are avoiding excess and adopting the rule of moderation. You still need calories to help you with processes such as maintaining your body heat.

In fact, you cannot completely remove energy from your body. If you do that, then you are violating the first rule of thermodynamics, which simply states that the internal work that is performed by the system has to equal the work that is done by that system. This means that you need just enough calories to ensure that you do not disrupt your body's normal functions or work.

Ketosis and autophagy cannot simply override or replace that.

Chapter 4: Surprising Benefits of One Meal a Day (OMAD)

When you have a culture saturated with the idea of excess, especially when it comes to food, then you have people trying to look for alternatives. When people become aware of the harmful effects of consuming too much of something, they realize that they should look for a method that might help them not just curb their habits, but bring their body into a better state.

At this point, people look to various dieting and fasting routines including your friendly neighborhood intermittent fasting.

At its core, intermittent fasting is beneficial to your body. You lose weight. You increase the rate at which fats are burned. You lower the levels of insulin and sugar in your bloodstream. You could even reverse the effects of type 2 diabetes.

With all of these advantages, intermittent fasting sounds like the ideal technique to focus on. While that may be true, intermittent fasting may not provide all the benefits that you might be seeking from the process. In other words, it is simply just not enough. Intermittent fasting has some incredible benefits when you look at the short-term, but it cannot guarantee benefits over a long period of time. And here is why.

In intermittent fasting, you are going without food anywhere from 12 to 16 hours. At the end of the period, you are going to eat food that benefits you. You are going to fill yourself with the right nutrients and the right amount of fats. You are ideally looking to lose as much weight as possible, remove harmful cells from your body, and live a long life with as many physical and mental benefits as you can possibly attain.

With intermittent fasting, you are not giving your body enough time to completely enter ketosis and bring about the process of autophagy. This is because, by the time the processes kick in, you have already provided food and nourishment to your body. You delay the processes slightly more.

This does not mean that intermittent fasting is not useful or does not work. It does! But we are looking to get your body into a healthier state of being through a much better method that sustains your health over a long period of time.

And is there such a method for you to use?

There is.

Let me introduce you to OMAD.

In OMAD fasting, you are aiming for a 23:1 ratio or a 20:4 ratio. What does this mean? Well, you are allowing your body between 20 and 23 hours every day to take advantage of the fasting process. You could be using the process for numerous reasons, maybe you aim to burn fat, improve your mental focus and attention, reduce your dependency on harmful foods, or simply help your body remove those compounds that are causing it harm. Whatever your reasons are when you begin to live on one meal a day you are taking your keto diet to the next level.

Fasting techniques such as OMAD boost your body by triggering stress response pathways that enhance the performance of your mitochondria (the organelle in the cell that is responsible for energy production), kick start the autophagy process, and improve the repair of DNA in your cells. OMAD also activates useful metabolic changes and reduces the risk of getting a chronic disease.

Apart from the above benefits, OMAD is known to increase your tolerance to hunger and allows your body to burn more fat for longer periods. OMAD also adds the benefit of lowering your blood sugar levels better than intermittent fasting. It increases the function of the insulin in your body. When you combine lowered blood sugar levels and improved insulin function, then you can reduce obesity much more effectively than any other form of fasting.

When you combine this with your keto diet, you are creating a method that helps you improve on the benefits that intermittent fasting can provide.

You are creating the ultimate form of fasting.

You are ready to be the Jedi knight of fasting.

Of course, there is much to learn before that so let us strap in. We are now going to find out just why OMAD is so good for us.

- For one, you are building a certain type of hormone called Human Growth Hormone, or HGH. This hormone serves plenty of purposes, but the benefit that we are most interested in at this point is the fact that HGH helps in building muscles. This is important to know because many people are of the opinion that OMAD has a negative impact on the development of muscles. According to the US National Library of Medicine National Institutes of Health, it doesn't. Not even close.

- Remember the inflammatory levels that we were talking about? Well, turns out that you can reduce those levels faster through this fasting method.

- And who can forget those nasty diseases? OMAD makes certain that you are reducing the risk of neurodegenerative diseases and it does so much better than intermittent fasting.

- Oh and the best part? OMAD increases the autophagy pathways in our body. What does this mean? You have better autophagy, leading to a better system for eradicating cells and proteins that your body does not require.

If intermittent fasting is the Bruce Banner of fasting, then having a single meal a day is like having the power of the Hulk. You are going to have so much more energy and the fasting itself is going to be so much more powerful and potent.

Then again, what does that mean? How can we translate the power and energy that you feel into benefits that you can see in your lifestyle? What are the changes that you are going to notice in your life that visibly show that your OMAD diet is working?

Here are some of those changes or improvements:

Increased Productivity

The initial shift to one meal a day is not without its challenges. But that is to be expected. You are making a big leap into another territory that gives you numerous benefits but also cuts back on a lot of the calories and carbs that you have been consuming so far. After successfully conquering the first phase of the diet, you are then going to notice changes in your ability. You might find your energy levels increasing. You are going to be more productive during the day.

Laser-Like Focus

Every meal that you are going to consume is going to have the right amount of energy and the right nutrients for your body. You are going to avoid any compounds that are going to have a negative effect on your life. Eventually, as you digest your food, you are going to send all that energy throughout your body, increasing your focus, attention span, and even brain activity. You are going to not just live better, but perform better!

Mental Clarity

If you have worked in an office setting, then you might be aware of your co-workers often talking about having lunch or making breakfast plans. Food is obviously an integral part of our lives. However, in many cases, it becomes a component that seeks to grab our attention at multiple times during the day. We might be engaged in an activity and might suddenly find thoughts of food swirling in our head. We might try and ignore those thoughts but we know that eventually, we are going to cave in to the temptation and order food or cook something for ourselves. OMAD helps you control those urges. You are getting everything you require in one meal so you do not feel the compulsion to grab a bite when you least expect it.

Chapter 5: Exercising Around OMAD

When you are adopting a healthy lifestyle, being active and having a plan to include exercises or workout sessions in your day becomes an essential part of that lifestyle. The scheduling or timing of your exercises can impact the outcome on your one meal a day plan, especially if you find yourself already managing your hunger. There are also many other components to take into consideration depending on the goals and objectives of your exercises or workouts.

Here is something you should make a note of, when your body enters a state of fasting it burns off the sugar it has stored and then moves on to the fat. It breaks down the fat and then converts it into ketones as a source of fuel for the body.

But why does this happen during a fasting state?

It has to do with insulin. When your body has received food or when you have entered a state of feeding, the levels of insulin increases in the body. Insulin is known to regulate the breakdown of fat and numerous research studies have shown that an increase in insulin levels has been shown to control fat metabolism by up to 22%.

During a fasting state, you are controlling the levels of insulin in your body which in turn increases the breakdown of fat.

Additionally, when you work out during fasting, you can start to see an improvement in an area you might not have thought of before, depression. That is right. Combine your workouts with the reduced levels of insulin and you can regulate your mental state much better than before. You are less likely to encounter sudden shifts in your mood or state of mind.

This, in turn, helps you keep your mind active and focused. Your brain spends less time dealing with the effects of depression and stress, which means that you are keeping it healthy.

Let us take a look at a few tips and common concerns about exercises and workouts while adopting an OMAD plan.

What to Consider

- Time your workouts. Do not exercise for periods longer than 60 minutes.

- Keep yourself hydrated. Ensure that you consume water before, during, and after your exercises.

- Your body is one of your best indicators. If you feel weak or nauseated during your workouts, then do not continue further. A recommendation would be to consult with your physician to adjust your food and workout schedules in a way that could benefit you greatly.

- If you are engaged in intense exercises or weight training, then having your one meal of the day after your workouts becomes important. Consider arranging your workout plans accordingly

- Take into consideration factors such as when you last ate, your age, whether or not you are pregnant, your medical history, whether you are taking any medications, your current fitness level, and even your body mass. These factors help you decide the right type of exercise for your OMAD plans.

- Make sure that you are consuming food that is high in protein and contains good fats. Include non-starchy vegetables in your diet. We are going to talk more about the diet that you need to follow during OMAD in the next chapter.

What to Avoid

- Working out for more than 60 minutes.

- Working out if you have a medical condition.

- Performing intense exercises when you have low blood sugar levels.

- Eating meals rich in carbohydrates as it could set the stage for frequent bouts of hunger.

- Working out in the mornings. Morning workouts are a common practice among many people as it allows them to utilize the remaining hours of the day to do other things. Exercising in the mornings can also be a common practice among those people who have certain work schedules or family obligations. However, while in the process of OMAD, you remain in a state of fasting until your eating period arrives later during the day. This can be a challenge mentally because you might end up waiting a long time before you eat.

Let us take an example to illustrate this. You have set your eating schedule anywhere between 3 pm to 7 pm (as people typically schedule their eating periods in the evening). If you work out in the morning at around 9 am, then you will end up waiting for another five to eight hours before you can actually have your meal. That might be rather uncomfortable. Waiting for your eating period to arrive can be challenging enough for you, but throw in your morning exercises and you will only increase your hunger.

So when exactly is the right time to work out during the OMAD process?

The ideal exercising time is just before you have your one meal.

Taking the above example, if you are planning to have your one meal at 5 pm, then you should ideally plan your workouts around 3 or 4 pm. What you are trying to do is keep at least an hour difference between the time you conclude exercising and the time you are about to have your meal.

Of course, some people may not be able to schedule their exercises only in the evenings. What if you only have time in the mornings? Is there a way you can still make use of an OMAD diet?

There is definitely a way. You can use any of the below liquids:

Water

You should especially aim to have mineral water. There is a reason for the word "mineral" to appear in the phrase as numerous minerals are added to the liquid. The percentage of minerals may vary from one mineral water to another, so make sure you read the label to pick out the one you prefer.

One of the unsung heroes in the list of components in mineral water is sulfates.

Sulfur is the eighth most common component of your body in terms of mass. Your body cannot utilize sulfates by directly consuming sulfur. For that reason, you need to consume foods that contain sulfate. Your solution? Mineral water.

Coffee

One of the biggest advantages of having coffee during an OMAD diet is its ability to control your appetite. Additionally, since you are fasting, the coffee tends to have an even greater effect, supplying your body with even more energy.

Caffeine also releases a neurotransmitter in the brain called dopamine. Dopamine plays a vital role in your emotional and mental well-being. This means that having coffee improves your mood, increases your focus, and improves your productivity.

Bone Broth

This is highly recommended in small doses. Research conducted on obese people has shown that their bodies contain large amounts of a type of bacteria called Firmicutes. The research has also shown that Firmicutes help with extracting high amounts of calories from food. When you drink bone broth, you also consume high amounts of a certain compound known as L-glutamine. One of the most important functions of L-glutamine is to lower the number of Firmicutes in the stomach, eventually aiding in weight loss.

There are people who might complete their workout during the afternoons. If you are one of those people, then worry not. There is a schedule you can follow as well. Instead of keeping your mealtime during the evening, try and adjust it to your workout schedule. For example, if you are going to work out at 1 pm then your one meal of the day should be scheduled anywhere between 2:30 pm to 3 pm, depending on the length of your workout session.

Another question that is asked frequently when it comes to fasting is about the intake of BCAA. People who are engaged in regular workouts are sometimes known to take branched-chain amino acid supplements. So does taking these supplements break your fast?

The short answer is, yes it does.

Essentially, BCAA's are supplements that contain numerous micronutrients. One of the main components of BCAA are amino acids and these amino acids contain fairly high doses of proteins. Which is why, whether you consume BCAAs in tablet or powder form, you are still taking in nutrients that you are supposed to gain from your single meal of the day.

Furthermore, BCAAs also contain calories. This calorie content upsets the balance that you are trying to attain through your OMAD plan. You might still require BCAA depending on the goals you are trying to achieve through your workout routines.

For example, you could be:

- Building muscle

- Performing weight training

- Preparing for a bodybuilding contest

- Training for a physically demanding and competitive sport or feat of endurance

In such cases, you might have to take in BCAA to provide you the type of results you are seeking. If you are simply aiming to lose weight and attain a healthier lifestyle, then you do not have to include BCAA as part of your food intake.

Optimal Cardiovascular Training on OMAD

What exactly is a cardiovascular training or exercise?

Cardiovascular exercise aims to increase your heart and breathing rate to moderate or intense levels for a specific time. Typically, fitness coaches recommend raising the heartbeat for about 10 minutes or more. However, we are not going to aim to keep the heart rate high for longer periods (remember, you are on an OMAD diet). Some of the more common forms of cardio activities people engage in are jogging, running, brisk walking, swimming, cycling, and rowing. If you are headed for the gym, then you might find numerous cardio machines that include the treadmill, gym cycles, stepping machine, and more.

For your cardiovascular training, here are the steps you can follow:

Warm Up and Stretching

Make sure you warm up to get your blood flowing. Warm-ups are like the lubricants added to vehicles to smoothen the engines, they relax your muscles and allow you to move your body without much resistance.

Begin by carrying out a warmup for roughly five to ten minutes. Keep the warm-up at a low intensity. You are only trying to prep your muscles for the session and gradually increase your heart rate.

Next, start performing activities that raise your heart rate to about 50 to 60% of its maximum rate. You can use any activity to perform your workout. You could even use the treadmill. If you are opting to run or walk, begin by running or walking at a relaxed pace that gets you to this heart rate. You should have a nice, quick heart rate going and still be able to talk about the last season of Game of Thrones with your friend.

Finally, time to stretch. Work on the muscles you will be focusing on in your workout. Warm them up and then utilize stretches to increase their flexibility. If there are special routines for the muscle group you are going to focus on during your workout, then take advantage of those routines.

Frequency of Exercises

As you are dieting, research into fitness has shown that performing cardiovascular exercises for 150 minutes every week is beneficial to your health. You need to take part in moderate-intensity exercises or activities. Make sure that you are spreading out the workout sessions throughout the week instead of clustering them too close together.

Here is a tip from the American College of Sports Medicine. They recommend that you carry out cardiovascular exercises roughly three to five days a week. They further suggest giving your body the time to build and repair the muscles. Therefore, you could carry out the exercises on alternate days.

Duration of Exercises

Finally, we arrive at the most important question: how long is too long? Well, when you are engaged in cardiovascular exercises, you should ideally aim for anywhere between 20 to 60 minutes, based on your capacity and your goals. You should keep your heart rate within the level of intensity that I mentioned earlier. Do not try to work out beyond the 60-minute mark or you might feel faint or dizzy.

The Benefits of Exercising with OMAD

Based on a study conducted by the Healthy Active Living and Obesity Research Group at the University of Ottawa in Canada, overweight people who performed just 150 minutes of low to moderate exercises on a weekly basis lived nearly 4 years longer than overweight people who did not have any exercise routines in their lives.

This study reveals a lot about the importance of exercise. When you combine this benefit of exercise with the longevity you are gaining through OMAD, you have a perfect combination of habits that you need to incorporate in your life. Your one meal diet and your workout routines complement each other wonderfully to give you a fulfilled life.

And the best part is? You do not have to engage in strenuous activities or high-intensity workouts. You just need to walk. In fact, as an alternative to working out at the gym, you could choose to enjoy the outdoors through a brisk walking session.

Men and women are encouraged to add regular exercises into their lives. While it is true that workouts affect men and women differently, the situation only occurs for high-intensity workouts. When you engage in a low to moderate intensity activities or workouts, then you are performing the same activity regardless of your gender.

For example, men can lift much quicker than women. Which is why women may often focus on other forms of exercises.

However, when you are walking briskly, jogging, or using the treadmill, it does not matter whether you are male or female, you can take advantage of the exercise.

Resistance

You can also take advantage of resistance exercises. When you perform any exercise to move your body against a source of resistance, then you are involved in strength or resistance training. You can add resistance to your body by moving your body against gravity or by using certain objects to create resistance. Examples of such objects could be dumbbells. Various machines at the gym also add resistance to your body.

Not many people are used to resistance workouts. It might take them a while to adapt to the changes that these workouts can cause to your muscles. If you are new to resistance exercises, then you can make use of certain programs to help you get started.

I recommend the basic program by Alexander Juan Antonio Cortes' Foundations Program to be ideal for your requirements. If you are interested in the workout, head over to his website or type this address into your browser - https://cortes.site/foundations-program/

Calisthenics

Another type of exercise that you can take advantage of during your OMAD diet is calisthenics. Simply put, calisthenics is bodyweight training. When you make any movement that makes use of your body weight and nothing else, then you are performing calisthenics.

Here are a few different types of workouts that you can incorporate in your daily life for various purposes.

No Equipment Calisthenics

You have to perform four cycles of the below workouts:

- Squats – 8

- Lunges – 8

- Push-ups – 8

- Laying Down Leg Raises – 8

- Plank - If you are a beginner to planks, then simply hold them for 30 seconds. Increase the time as you improve.

- Pike Push-ups – 8

- Mountain Climbers – As many as possible (you can stick to about 20 climbers for each leg when you are starting out).

Basic Beginner Workout

You have to perform four cycles of the below workouts:

- Close Hands Chin Ups – 7

- Pull-ups – 5

- Dips – 6

- Push-ups – 15

- Laying Down Leg Raises – 8

- Jump Squats – 9

Fat Removal Workout

You have to perform four cycles of the below workouts:

- Run – 100 meters

- Dips – 5

- Jumping Jacks – 45 seconds

- Push-ups – 8

- Mountain climbers – 30 seconds

- Planks – 15 seconds

When you are carrying out the above exercises, make sure you schedule them on alternate days. Let us take an example of a schedule. Let us assume that you have chosen to work on the Basic Beginner Workout. Your schedule could look like this:

- Monday: Workout

- Tuesday: Rest Day

- Wednesday: Workout

- Thursday: Rest Day

- Friday: Workout

- Saturday: Workout

- Sunday: Rest Day

You can also combine different exercises to attain various results. For example, you could create a schedule such as the below:

- Monday: Basic Beginner Workout

- Tuesday: No Equipment Calisthenics

- Wednesday: Rest Day

- Thursday: Fat Removal Workout

- Friday: Rest Day

- Saturday: Basic Beginner Workout/Fat Removal Workout/ No Equipment Calisthenics (alternate between the three every week)

- Sunday: Rest Day

You can modify the above routine as you see fit. The idea is to make sure that you are giving your body the exercise it deserves along with your OMAD diet. This helps in creating a complete benefit package for your body.

Make sure that you are comfortable with the workouts. If you feel like you are on the verge of losing consciousness, then do not push yourself to continue further. Remember that you are giving your body a healthy routine. You are not trying to punish it.

But with all the talk of workouts, is there something you can take to make the most out of your workout sessions?

It turns out there is.

The use of apple cider vinegar (ACV) is not something that arose recently. It has been used for thousands of years in cooking. Over the years, it began to gain popularity as a natural remedy for numerous disorders and ailments. In fact, just head over to your local store and you might just spot the number of apple cider vinegar brands that are now lining up the shelves. So why has this mixture gained a boost in popularity in recent years?

Here is one reason, the intake of the vinegar is considered to provide your body with plenty of benefits when combined with exercise including weight loss, lowered blood sugar levels, prevention of diabetes and more.

The best part of having apple cider vinegar is that it does not compromise on flavor. Many people have remarked on the fact that the vinegar is actually rather tasty.

So how can you combine ACV with your workouts? Is there anything else you should be adding to your intake of ACV?

Let us take an example. We have just discovered that ACV helps with weight loss. Imagine if you combine ACV with the Fat Removal Workout. You are not only going to enjoy the benefits of weight loss through your workout, but you are going to ensure that you manage your weight by consuming ACV.

While you are combining ACV with your exercises, you can add in another complimentary ingredient to the mix: creatine.

As you are engaged in managing your weight and creating a healthier lifestyle for yourself, you might need a source of energy for your workouts.

Why is creatine so useful? For one, it helps your muscles produce more energy. This means that you can work out without getting tired really fast. Additionally, creatine is a popular supplement for adding muscle mass. This means that you are not just maintaining a healthy routine, but you are improving your muscles as well.

Here are some of the other ways that creatine is useful for your body:

Supports High-Intensity Exercises

Creatine plays a vital role in the production of adenosine triphosphate, or ATP. Now, what is so special about this ATP? It actually does sound like the name of a medicinal drug. Thankfully, it isn't. However, it is an important component in your body. In fact, it is your body's energy source. When your body breaks down ATP, the process releases energy that is utilized by the tissues and various other parts of your body.

Fights Neurological Diseases

One of the reasons why neurological diseases spread really fast is because of the low levels of phosphocreatine in your brain. This reduces the energy levels supplied to your brain and weakens it. In research conducted on mice with Huntington's disease, adding creatine helped in restoring the brain's phosphocreatine levels. This improved brain functions and returned the brain to nearly 72% of its original state (or its pre-Huntington's disease state)! That is an incredible result and goes to show how just the absence one chemical can create such a drastic effect on the body. It also shows why creatine is not just a muscle booster. It is a powerful compound used for various processes in the body.

Brain Functions

As we are already focused on the region of the brain, let us continue to show how creatine further enhances the region. This is why meat is important.

Wait a minute. That was a random fact just throw in to show support to the meat eaters. Vegetarian for life!

That's not it. In fact, I wholly support a wholesome vegetarian meal. However, the fact remains and science backs it up: meat is the best source of creatine. This is why vegetarians experience low levels of creatine in their bodies.

Does that mean you have to now give up your vegetarian diet and start sinking your teeth into some steak?! Not exactly. What you should be doing is adding creatine supplements to your diet to provide you with the necessary amount of the compound. In fact, in one study made on creatine, simply adding supplements that included the compound in the diet of vegetarians resulted in up to a 50% improvement in the intelligence and memory scores of the participants, showing an overall improvement in brain functions. Of course, if you are consuming meat, we are going to ensure that you consume the right meat as part of your OMAD diet. After all, what you eat plays a vital role in providing you with the right nutrients.

So imagine this scenario: you consume creatine to ensure that you have the energy for your exercises. You perform low- to moderate-intensity exercises to keep your body fit while you are dieting. You also add in ACV to ensure that you maintain your weight while throwing in some additional benefits such as prevention of diseases and lowering of your blood sugar levels. Sounds like a pretty potent combination, doesn't it?

And that is exactly why you should be adding creatine to your exercise routine along with a steady

Jason Michaels *&* Thomas Hawthorn

supply of ACV. It helps you maintain muscle while you are in a state of fasting.

Chapter 6: Foods You Think Are Keto-Friendly, But Aren't

We have all been there. We are certain that a particular food is definitely meant for our keto diet, only to discover that we have been wrong about that food. Trust me, I have encountered those scenarios quite a few times.

We are inundated with so much information that separating the wheat from the chaff becomes a challenging prospect. This becomes true when you have many sources of information claiming that they are backed up by science when they are in fact, just theories and guesses.

Most foods that you encounter in your life have carbs. Even certain types of meat, vegetables, and nuts contain some amount of carbs.

In fact, have you heard of the phrase "hidden carbs"?

You see, many dieters switch to low-carb diets each year. They are ready to give up a lot of foods such as bread, pasta, and rice. They decide to dial back on numerous fruits. They cut down on previous habits. Once all that is done, they believe that they are now of a journey to experience a low-carb diet! They have succeeded in creating the perfect plan for themselves!

Yet for all their efforts, they have no idea of some of the sources of carbs. They might consume these foods, thinking that they are now safe within the boundaries of a low-carb diet.

If only they knew.

Here are some foods that actually have more carbs than you might have been aware of:

Low-Fat Foods

Have you ever walked by a supermarket aisle and spotted foods like dressings, peanut butter, and other items with the tag "low-fat"? Sounds tempting, doesn't it? It is like your prayers have been answered! Finally, you can enjoy some delicious food without worrying about any fattening ingredients.

Here is the reality of the situation. To ensure that the flavors of the low-fat products are not lost, food manufacturers generally replace fat with sugar. This increases the carb count rather than lowering it.

Liquid Eggs

In a world where you can get a canned or packaged version of so many foods (in fact, I actually spotted a pre-packed Indian butter chicken, how is that even possible?!), one of the ideas that has gained a fair amount of popularity in recent times is liquid eggs. You might have noticed containers of the stuff. All you have to do is pour them into a pan and you are ready to start cooking.

The reality? Not only do container eggs or liquid eggs contain certain ingredients and compounds that aren't usually found in an egg - such as xanthan gum – they are also infused with high fructose corn syrup (of course they are). Manufacturers are required to list the contents of their foods. But when you actually head over to products that contain corn syrup, you might notice something rather peculiar.

There is no mention of corn syrup on the label!

But how?!

Does this mean that you can now sue the company and win a million dollar lawsuit, after which you can finally retire on an island of your choice with a martini in your hand?! Quick, time to call in the best lawyers in the city!

Not so fast.

The reason why corn syrup is missing from the label is that it appears under another name: maltodextrin.

Pretty cunning isn't it?

Sauces

If your plate is covered with lots of healthy vegetables, then that is awesome! But if those vegetables are covered in a not-so-conservative amount of gravy and sauces, then you are about to consume a lot of carbs.

Restaurants need to sell their food. They need to make sure that the flavor is just right. Which is why, many of these outlets use sugar or flour, and both items contain a not-so-healthy dose of carbs. Before you know it, you are slurping away incredible amounts of carbs into your body. Yum!

Certain Vegetables

Oh yes. You might not have expected vegetables to turn up on this list but certain varieties of these foods actually contain a rather large amount of carbs. Brussel sprouts, broccoli, and squash are some examples that have high carbs but are still included in the diets of many people. This is because people are not actually aware of how many carbs these vegetables supply to you.

Want to know some of the other vegetables that are high in carbs?

Get ready because some of the items on this list might very well surprise you.

- Black-eyed peas

- Carrots

- Garbanzo beans

- Green peas

- Lima beans

- Parsnips

- Pinto beans

- Potato

- Pumpkin

- Sweet potato

- White beans

That is right. Carrots have high carbs too.

In fact, you might have been eating the vegetables in the above list and been confident of the fact that you are on the path to a healthy diet.

So what vegetables are actually safe to consume? Is there nothing that you can eat?

The answer is simple: you have a lot of options. In fact, you could be spoilt for choice when it comes to having vegetables with low-carbs. The trick is to identify them.

Spinach, mushroom, onion, asparagus, zucchini, eggplant, tomato, cabbage, peppers, and kale are just some of the examples of low-carb vegetables.

Once you begin to separate vegetables based on their carbs, you have a better idea of how you can manage your diet.

Chapter 7: 28 –Day OMAD Autophagy Meal Plan

There is a reason why OMAD works so well.

When you have one meal a day, you are storing fat only when you are feeding. This is because when you eat, insulin gets released into your bloodstream to regulate your blood sugar levels. Any extra sugar is then used for the muscles, liver, or stored as fat. When you are not eating, insulin does not get released and the aforementioned process does not occur.

If we actually start to think about it, the whole idea of having three or four meals a day does not sound practical. You are releasing insulin every time you eat. You are storing more and more fat in your body.

Nobody wants more fat.

Except perhaps your wallet. A fat wallet is a good sign.

But we are talking about your body so we are going to just use the required amount of fat.

And how do we do that?

We start with a 28-day OMAD Autophagy meal plan.

Remember, you are supposed to eat this meal anywhere between 5 pm to 7 pm.

Before we delve into some delicious recipes that you can enjoy during your OMAD diet, here are some important points that you should think about.

Caffeine

Caffeine is addictive and many of us consume way too much.

Most of us like to enjoy a nice cup of joe. That is okay. What is not okay is depending heavily on coffee to receive your energy. This is because our dependency becomes our weakness. We start taking too much of it and that ends up affecting our sleep patterns, which in turn begins to affect our fasting plan. When we drink coffee, we should aim to have a maximum of two cups a day. We should try not to have coffee beyond the 2 pm mark. Doing so might affect our sleep. While it is true that each person tolerates caffeine differently, it is not prudent to experiment just to get an extra cup of coffee in a day. Remember, you are heading towards a healthier lifestyle. Why ruin it?

Treats

Right, we all love to enjoy treats. And it becomes especially tempting to fall prey to your cravings when you are on a diet. But do not worry! I have included some incredible treats for you to enjoy. I also have a cappuccino treat waiting for you as well! So keep off those chocolate brownies for now.

Bread

People are so dependent on bread that they do not think twice about how many carbs they are consuming. It just becomes a natural part of their lives. In the following recipes, I have avoided bread to the best of my extent. Some people claim that having a single piece of bread occasionally is all right. Remember this, each person's body functions in a different way. You do not want to ruin your plan by trying to see if a single piece of bread will affect your body or not.

Sticking to the Schedule

I understand that people have commitments. You have to focus on different areas of your life and they might interrupt your OMAD plan. However, what is important to note is that there is no easy path to achieving good health. Want to gain weight? Pop some Cheetos and Nutella. Want to gain muscles? Sweat every day at the gym.

You see the difference there, right?

That is why I recommend that you try and stick to the plan as much as possible. It is true that the initial phase is going to be difficult. In fact, those who have ventured out to the gym know that the first few days involve quite a few muscle pains and cramps. Starting this diet will be no different.

The Grass Is Greener (and Healthier) on the Other Side

Most people find the first week or so a challenging phase of the plan.

When your body begins to detox and cleanse, it may lead to headaches and lack of energy. You might decide that this plan is not worth it. But as I mentioned in the previous section, no matter what activity, course, plan, or sessions you choose to live a better life, you will always have to go through the tough introductory part.

There is, however, a way you can minimize some of the discomfort you might feel. Make sure you are rehydrating yourself with at least 2 liters of water.

Once you have passed the initial stages of the plan, the rest of the way is a walk in the park.

Note: As this is your only meal for the day, 4 "servings" is the serving size for 1 person. So your average calorie intake will be between 1600-1800 calories per day. If you require more (use this online tool to calculate your needs) https://www.active.com/fitness/calculators/bmr - then you can increase serving size as necessary.

Your OMAD Shopping List

Here are some of the things you should be shopping for when you hit the local supermarket. Do note that as you go through each recipe, you might get a better idea of the kind of ingredients that you might want to purchase.

Fats & Oils

Try to get your fat from natural sources like meat and nuts. Supplement with saturated and monounsaturated fats like coconut oil, butter, and olive oil.

Protein

Try to stick with organic, pasture-raised and grass-fed meat where possible. Most meats don't have added sugar in them, so they can be consumed in moderate quantity. Remember that too much protein on a ketogenic diet is not a good thing.

Vegetables

It does not matter whether you pick fresh or frozen vegetables. Stick with above ground vegetables, leaning toward leafy/green items.

Dairy

Most dairy is fine, but make sure to buy full-fat dairy items. Harder cheeses typically have fewer carbs.

Nuts and Seeds

In moderation, nuts and seeds can be used to create some fantastic textures. Try to use fattier nuts like macadamias and almonds.

Beverages

Stay simple and stick to mostly water. You can flavor it if needed with stevia-based flavorings or lemon/lime juice.

Day 1

Summer Shrimp Salad

Tomatoes, thyme, and shrimp make this not just a healthy meal but one that pleases the visual senses!

Serving Size

4 servings

Ingredients

1 ¼ pounds Raw Shrimps

3 large tomatoes (chopped)

1 medium-sized English cucumber

10 sprigs fresh thyme

¼ cup extra-virgin olive oil

4 cloves garlic (crushed)

¼ teaspoon salt

¼ teaspoon ground pepper

¼ cup lemon juice

½ cup fresh basil (chopped)

Extra basil for garnish

Instructions

- Begin by preheating the oven to 350°F.

- Mix the shrimp with the thyme and garlic on a rimmed baking sheet. Add oil and mix again. Sprinkle the mixture with salt and pepper.

- Pop the mix into the oven and bake until you see the shrimp turning firm and pink: ideally for 8 – 10 minutes.

- Take out the mix and add your lemon juice. Stir the juice into the mix.

- Add in the tomatoes, cucumber, and basil and gently stir again.

- Next, transfer the salad into a bowl.

- Garnish it with basil to complete the meal prep.

Nutrition Information (per serving)

- Calories – 410 calories

- Fat – 15 grams

- Carbs – 8 grams

- Protein – 31 grams

Day 2

Grilled Fish Peperonata

Grilled fish with some peppers? Yes to the flavor please! If you like, you can prepare the peperonata in advance and then reheat it again when you are grilling the fish.

Serving Size

4 Servings

Ingredients

1 ½ pounds skinned swordfish, amberjack, or mahi-mahi

3 garlic cloves (sliced)

1 medium-sized red onion (thinly sliced)

8 cups bell peppers of any color (thinly sliced)

¼ cup fennel (thinly sliced)

1 teaspoon fresh oregano (chopped)

1 teaspoon fresh thyme (chopped)

1 teaspoon paprika

½ teaspoon kosher salt

2 tablespoons sherry vinegar

2 tablespoons extra-virgin olive oil

Additional extra-virgin olive oil for grilling

Pinch of crushed red pepper

¼ cup parsley or basil for garnish

Instructions

- Heat 2 tablespoons of extra-virgin olive oil in a large pot over medium heat. Toss in your garlic, crushed red pepper, and cook. Stir occasionally (for about 2 to 3 minutes) until you can smell the fragrance and the garlic begins to show a brown color. Add the onion and continue stirring (for around 5 minutes) until the onions become soft.

- Add the oregano, paprika, and thyme.

- Add in the bell peppers and stir for around 10 seconds. Reduce the heat to a low degree and continue to cook the ingredients for about 15 to 20 minutes. Stir occasionally.

- Add the vinegar into the mix and cook for around 2 minutes more.

- Set the mixture aside and turn to the grill. Preheat the grill to a medium-high temperature. Use a brush and apply the oil to the fish, brushing gently. Sprinkle the fish with salt.

- Next, use the brush to oil the grill.

- Place the fish on the grill. Allow it to grill for around 5 minutes or until the flesh is opaque and then flip it over. Grill the other side for about 3 minutes or until you notice the opaque consistency.

- Take out the fish and use a cutting board to chop the fish into 4 pieces.

- Take out your plate. Place the peperonata on it (try and decorate your plate with it).

- Place your fish over the peperonata.

- Sprinkle with parsley or basil for garnish.

Nutrition Information (per serving)

- Calories – 420 calories

- Fat – 25 grams

- Carbs – 8.5 grams

- Protein – 32 grams

Day 3

Cuban Stromboli

A Cuban sandwich delight that adds the right amount of healthy ingredients and flavor! Plus, it has cheese.

Serving Size

6 servings

Ingredients

5 ounces pizza dough (whole wheat)

4 slices of Swiss cheese (preferably thin slices)

3 slices ham

3 slices turkey

4 slices salami

1 pickle sliced lengthwise

1 egg yolk (preferably large)

1 teaspoon water

Sesame seeds

Yellow mustard

Instructions

- Start off by preheating the oven to 450°F.

- Use a clean surface and lightly flour it. Roll out your pizza dough on the surface. Cut out rectangles measuring 12 inches by 6 inches.

- Add a layer of salami, ham, pickle, turkey, and Swiss cheese for each rectangular slice.

- Roll the slice along the long side of the rectangle. Ensure that the roll is tight.

- Take out your baking tray and cover it with a baking sheet.

- Place your rolls on the baking sheet.

- Use a knife to cut a few slits on the top of each roll.

- Take your egg yolk and add it to a bowl. Add the water into it. Whisk the mixture thoroughly.

- Use a brush to apply the yolk and water mixture on the top of the rolls.

- Sprinkle the rolls with sesame seeds.

- Pop the tray into the oven and bake it for not more than 20 minutes or until the rolls turn golden brown.

- Finally, serve the rolls with mustard if you like.

Nutrition Information (per serving)

- Calories – 276 calories

- Fat – 6 grams

- Carbs – 5 grams

- Protein – 4 grams

Day 4

Grilled Smoky Flank Steak

Who doesn't love a nice juicy steak? What? You thought this book was going to exclude steak? Not likely!

Serving Size

4 servings

Ingredients

Jason Michaels & Thomas Hawthorn

5 pounds flank steak (trimmed)

1 ½ teaspoons smoked paprika

1 ½ teaspoons white vinegar

½ teaspoon ground chipotle chili

½ teaspoon salt

1 teaspoon brown sugar

¼ teaspoon ground pepper

¼ teaspoon garlic powder

Instructions

- Preheat your grill to a medium to medium-high temperature.

- In a small bowl, mix together the oil, chipotle chili, vinegar, garlic powder, paprika, salt, and pepper.

- One the ingredients are mixed well, use a brush and apply them over your steak. Alternatively, you can use your hands to rub the mixture over your steak. I prefer using your hands as it ensures that mixture is applied really well.

- Place your steak on the grill.

- Insert a thermometer into the thickest part of the steak.

- Grill until the thermometer reads about 120°F for a medium-rare steak.

- Once done, flip over the steak and grill again. Ideally, you should be grilling for 3 to 5 minutes per side.

- Take out the steak and place it on a plate. Allow it to rest for about 5 minutes

- Slice into 4 pieces.

Nutrition Information (per serving)

- Calories – 350 calories

- Fat – 12 grams

- Carbs – 2 grams

- Protein – 23 grams

Day 5

Crispy Salmon Caprese Salad

Another day, another exciting salad for you to eat. This time, we are jumping away from shrimp and entering the salmon territory.

Serving Size

4 servings

Ingredients

1 salmon fillet - large

1 cucumber (chopped) - large

1 cup cherry tomatoes (chopped in half)

1/2 cup fresh basil leaves (chopped)

4 tablespoons extra-virgin olive oil

1 tablespoon balsamic vinegar

½ teaspoon salt

½ teaspoon pepper

225 grams baby mozzarella balls

Instructions

- Let us get the salmon ready first. Take out a skillet and place it over medium-high heat. Allow it to heat up a little bit.

- Add 1 tablespoon of olive oil into the skillet. To spread the oil evenly, take out the skillet and gently rotate your wrist. Do not keep the skillet away from the flame for too long.

- Place the salmon skin side down into the skillet. Allow the salmon to cook for about 5 minutes. Turn over the salmon and cook the other side for about 3 to 4 minutes.

- Take out the salmon from the skillet. Remove the skin.

- In a large bowl, add tomatoes, cucumber, mozzarella balls, basil, and the remaining 3 tablespoons of olive oil. Mix well.

- Chop the salmon into small pieces and add them to the bowl. Mix again.

- Add salt and pepper to taste if you prefer. Add in the balsamic vinegar as well.

Nutrition Information (per serving)

- Calories – 407 calories

- Fat – 28 grams

- Carbs – 6 grams

- Protein – 29 grams

Day 6

Chicken Meatball Soup

A nice warm soup to add in a level of comfort after a hard day of fasting? Do I hear a "where do I get one?" Well, in your kitchen of course!

Serving Size

4 servings

Ingredients for the meatballs

2 chicken breasts, chopped

2 cloves garlic

2 tablespoon parsley (chopped)

1 tablespoon tomato puree

½ brown onion (chopped)

½ teaspoon salt

½ teaspoon pepper

1 tablespoon extra-virgin olive oil

Ingredients for the Soup

½ brown onion (chopped)

2 celery sticks, preferably medium (chopped)

2 carrots, preferably medium (chopped)

4 cups low-sodium chicken broth

1 teaspoon dried thyme

½ teaspoon salt

½ teaspoon pepper

1 tablespoon extra-virgin olive oil

Instructions

We'll start with the meatballs.

- Start by preheating the oven to 390°F.

- To make the meatballs, place all the ingredients for the meatballs inside a food processor and blitz them. Make sure that they appear well-combined.

- Begin creating rolls of meatballs, ideally with your hands.

- You should have no more than 20 meatballs, depending on the size.

- Take out a baking tray and cover it with a baking sheet.

- Take out a brush and apply the extra-virgin olive oil on the meatballs.

- Pop the tray into the oven and bake it for about 20 minutes or until you notice the meatballs turning a golden brown color.

While the meatballs are baking, time to prepare the soup.

- Take out a pan and heat at a medium-low setting. Add in the olive oil. Toss in the celery, onion, and carrots and stir them for about 4 to 5 minutes or until you see them softening.

- Add in the broth and the thyme. Season. Bring the soup to a boil and then reduce the heat to medium. Let the soup simmer for about 15 minutes.

- Add the kale into the soup and let cook for about 1 to 2 minutes or until it softens.

- Finally, add in your chicken meatballs.

Nutrition Information (per serving)

- Calories – 357 calories

- Fat – 19 grams

- Carbs – 6 grams

- Protein – 32 grams

Day 7

Green Shakshouka

Shakshouka is such a comfort food for many people. Turn it green with some spinach and feta and you have created a delicious and healthy meal to end your fast!

Serving Size

6 servings

Ingredients

12 ounces chard (stemmed properly and chopped)

12 ounces spinach (stemmed properly and chopped)

6 eggs, preferably large

2 garlic cloves (chopped)

2 tablespoons unsalted butter

1 onion (chopped), preferably large

1 small serrano pepper (thinly sliced)

½ cup low-sodium chicken broth

½ cup feta cheese

4 tablespoons extra-virgin olive oil

1 tablespoon balsamic vinegar

¼ teaspoon salt

¼ teaspoon pepper

Instructions

- Place a skillet over medium heat. Allow it to heat up a little.

- Once the skillet is hot, add in the oil and allow it to heat as well.

- Add in the onion and begin cooking. Stir in as frequently as possible for about 7 to 8 minutes, until you begin to notice the onions turning translucent and soft. However, do not allow the onions to brown.

- Add the spinach and the chard into the skillet. The best way to add them is by handfuls. Take a handful of chard and spinach, place it into the skillet and then repeat the process. Cook them until you notice them becoming wilted, which typically happens in about 5 minutes.

- Add in your balsamic vinegar, serrano, garlic, salt, and pepper. Stir the ingredients together for about 2 to 4 minutes until you notice the garlic softening.

- Bring in the broth and the butter to the mixture. Continue stirring until the butter melts.

- Next, take your eggs and crack them over the vegetables.

- Place a cover over the skillet and then turn the heat to medium-low. Cook the shakshouka for about 3 to 5 minutes until you see the eggs turn white.

- Finally, remove the skillet from heat and sprinkle it with cheese. Place the cover over the skillet again and allow it to rest for about 2 minutes before serving.

Nutrition Information (per serving)

- Calories – 296 calories

- Fat – 23 grams

- Carbs – 5 grams

- Protein – 11 grams

Day 8

Crispy Artichokes

Imagine this, delicious crispy artichokes placed on top of smooth labneh. Boy that is one way to sit down, relax, and enjoy a meal that just brings a smile to your face. You might have to start preparing the recipe in the morning or at least a week in advance as a part of the recipe relies on refrigeration. I would recommend that you start a week in advance.

Serving Size

6 servings

Ingredients

4 cups plain yogurt. I highly recommend the whole-milk variety. Other forms of yogurt have high carbs.

4 cups canola oil

4 cloves garlic

3 tablespoons lemon juice

2 cans of artichoke hearts. Make sure you rinse them, then halve them, and finally set them out to dry

¼ cup parsley (chopped)

Instructions

- Firstly, you will need a sieve and a bowl. The bowl should be deep enough that if you place the sieve inside the bowl, there are at least 3 inches of space between the bottom of the sieve and the bowl. Ensure that the sieve has a diameter of at least 7 inches or bigger.

- Next, place 4 layers of cheesecloth into the sieve. Make sure that you line each cheesecloth properly. Then place the sieve into the bowl.

- In another bowl, add the yogurt and pour the lemon juice into it. Whisk them well. Transfer the yogurt mixture from the second bowl into the sieve. Make sure that you get as much of the yogurt into the sieve as possible.

- Now you have to refrigerate until the yogurt is thick and you notice at least 1 cup of liquid has drained into the bowl. As mentioned earlier, you can choose to refrigerate it starting early in the morning or up to 1 week in advance.

- Once you have refrigerated the labneh for the recommended duration, take out the sieve and discard the liquid.

- Transfer the sieve into a medium bowl.

- Add ¼ tablespoon of salt and stir well.

- Now it is time to work on the artichokes. Pour the oil into a large saucepan and bring it to medium-high heat. Start frying your artichokes for about 2 to 3 minutes until they turn golden brown and crispy.

- Transfer the artichokes to a medium-sized bowl (yes, this recipe is going to require quite a few bowls). Add in the garlic, parsley, and the remaining salt.

- Finally, take the labneh and spread it over a plate. Add the crispy artichokes on top.

- If you prefer, you can serve the dishes with a couple of lemon wedges.

Nutrition Information (per serving)

- Calories – 323 calories

- Fat – 26 grams

- Carbs – 13 grams

- Protein – 10 grams

Day 9

Bacon with Sautéed Radishes

We had steak. Now it is time to introduce some bacon into your diet. One of the best aspects of this dish is that it is easy to make and even if you do not like radishes, you might just find them enjoyable after this meal.

Serving Size

4 servings

Ingredients

12 ounces radishes (quartered)

6 shallots (quartered), preferably medium

3 slices bacon (chopped)

2 teaspoons garlic (finely chopped)

1 teaspoon fresh thyme (chopped)

1 ½ tablespoons cider vinegar

1 ½ teaspoons unsalted butter

¼ teaspoon salt

¼ teaspoon pepper

Instructions

- Place a skillet over medium-high heat.

- Once the skillet is hot, place the bacon strips into the skillet. Flip the bacon occasionally for about 5 to 6 minutes until they turn crispy.

- Cover a plate with a paper towel. Transfer the bacon onto the plate. Make sure that you leave the drippings in the skillet.

- Add in the shallots and the radishes. Cook them for about 2 to 3 minutes until they are charred slightly on one side. Once you notice the char, continue to cook until they turn brown all over. Make sure you do not char them too much at this point.

- Throw in your thyme and garlic and stir.

- Add the salt and pepper and continue to stir for about 1 minute until you smell the fragrance.

- Take the skillet off the heat and then add in the butter and vinegar.

- Mix everything together well.

- Finally, add the thyme as a garnish.

Nutrition Information (per serving)

- Calories – 285 calories

- Fat – 12 grams

- Carbs – 9 grams

- Protein – 5 grams

Day 10

Cappuccino Chia Macadamia Pudding

When you deserve to enjoy a nice treat, you can simply make this little delight. Did I also mention that it is actually healthy?

Serving Size

6 servings

Ingredients

1 cup chia seeds

½ cup espresso

3 cups and 3 tablespoons macadamia or almond milk (make sure you get the unsweetened variety)

1 teaspoon vanilla extract (sugar-free)

1 teaspoon cacao powder or cinnamon

Stevia to taste

Instructions

Starting with the coffee

- Add ⅔ cup of chia seeds to a blender and grind them into a powder (alternately, keep the seeds whole for more texture).

- Next, pour in 2 cups and 2 tablespoons of your macadamia or almond milk as well as the ½ cup of espresso.

- Blend it all together and taste, add stevia if desired.

- Pour into your cup till the cup is ⅔ full and cool the mix in the fridge.

Continuing with the vanilla topping

- Clean the blender then add in ⅓ cup chia seeds, the remaining 1 cup and 1 tablespoon of macadamia or almond milk, 1 teaspoon vanilla extract, 1 teaspoon of cacao powder. Blend until smooth.

- Add stevia to taste, if desired.

- Pour this on top of the coffee and cool in the fridge for at least an hour prior to serving.

- You can sprinkle additional cacao powder on top right before serving to give it some extra flavor.

Nutrition Information (per serving)

- Calories – 151 calories

- Fat – 9.7 grams

- Carbs – 2.4 grams

- Protein – 5.8 grams

Day 11

Tomato Dolma

Time to have a few stuffed vegetables. Especially if the stuffing is ground beef and eggplants.

Serving Size

12 servings

Ingredients

12 tomatoes, preferably medium sized

3 tablespoons bulgur

2 tablespoons extra-virgin olive oil

2 cloves garlic

1 eggplant, preferably large

1 onion, preferably medium

1 teaspoon ground cumin

1 pound ground beef

1 teaspoon salt

½ teaspoon pepper

¼ cup fresh mint (chopped)

Instructions

- Start off by preheating the grill on high heat.

- Next, use a fork to prick an eggplant. Now slowly grill it, making sure you turn occasionally. Grill for 10 to 15 minutes until you notice the eggplant turn tender and charred. Transfer to a plate to cool. Once cool, peel the eggplant and transfer it to a bowl. Add the juices from the plate into the bowl and mash the eggplant. Let it sit for 10 minutes.

- Next, preheat your oven to 400°F. Take out a baking dish and lightly coat it with cooking spray.

- Take your tomatoes and cut off their tops. Do not dispose of the tops as we will require them later. Remove the inside of the tomato with a spoon.

- Take the insides of the tomato and place them in a blender. Add oil, ¼ teaspoon salt, and pepper and then blend it until it becomes a puree. Take the puree and spread it inside the baking dish.

- Use some of the remaining salt to sprinkle the insides of the tomatoes.

- Return to the eggplant. Add the ground beef, garlic, onion, bulgur, cumin, and the remaining salt and pepper into the eggplant. Mix well. Take the mixture and stuff the tomatoes with it.

- Replace the cut-off tops of the tomatoes.

- Place the tomatoes in the baking dish, use foil to cover the dish.

- Place the dish in the oven and bake for about 15 minutes. Next, take off the foil and continue baking for another 30 or 35 minutes.

- Take out the dish and sprinkle the tomatoes with mint.

Nutrition Information (per serving)

- Calories – 131 calories

- Fat – 9 grams

- Carbs – 3 grams

- Protein – 9 grams

Day 12

Low-Carb Walnut and Zucchini Salad

Walnut and zucchini are both healthy foods. Combine them and you have a healthy salad to finish your day.

Serving Size

4 servings

Ingredients for the Dressing

2 tablespoons olive oil

2 teaspoons lemon juice

1 garlic clove

¼ cup low-carb mayonnaise

½ teaspoon salt

¼ teaspoon chili powder

Ingredients for the Salad

4 ounces arugula lettuce

2 zucchini

1 head of Romaine lettuce

1 tablespoon olive oil

¾ cup chopped walnuts or pecans

¼ cup finely chopped fresh chives or scallions

¼ teaspoon salt

¼ teaspoon pepper

Instructions

- Take out a small bowl. Toss in all the ingredients necessary to make the dressing and whisk them together well. Set aside the dressing so that the flavors develop. In the meantime, turn your attention to the salad.

- Cut the zucchini into halves length-wise and remove the seeds. Next, chop the zucchini halves, preferably into half-inch pieces.

- Take out a frying pan and pour the olive oil in it. Allow the oil to heat up over medium heat until you see it simmering.

- Place your chopped zucchini in the pan. Season it with salt and pepper.

- Sauté the zucchini until it turns a light brown color.

- Trim and cut the salad. Place the romaine, arugula, and chives in a large bowl.

- Next, cut the lettuces and mix them into the large bowl.

- Add in your zucchini and mix well.

- Take out your nuts and roast them in the same pan you used to prepare your zucchini. Season lightly with salt and pepper.

- Toss them into the bowl with the zucchini and mix well.

- Finally, drizzle your salad with the dressing.

Nutrition Information (per serving)

- Calories – 456 calories

- Fat – 54 grams

- Carbs – 7 grams

- Protein – 8 grams

Day 13

Low-carb Tartlets with Caramelized Onion and Brie

These little delights remind you of mini pies, minus all the carbs and calories!

Serving Size

12 tartlets

Ingredients for the Crust

1 batch of keto pie crust

Ingredients for the Cheese filling

2 medium red onions (thinly sliced)

2 tablespoons extra-virgin olive oil

2 tablespoons balsamic vinegar (30 ml)

12 small wedges brie cheese

¼ cup fresh herbs such as thyme or rosemary

½ teaspoon sea salt, for taste

Instructions

- Preheat the oven to 355°F.

- Next, take out a frying pan and place it over medium heat. Pour a little olive oil into it and bring it to a simmer.

- Toss in your onions, and cook. Stir occasionally until you see the onions soften.

- Bring down the heat to low. Add your vinegar and salt, and continue cooking. Stir occasionally. Wait until the onions have caramelized.

- While the onions are becoming caramelized, take out 12 muffin tins. Grease them inside and press your pie crust into these muffin tins.

- Once done, pop them into the oven and bake for about 10 minutes. Remove the pie crusts from the oven and allow them to cool at room temperature, ideally for about 5 minutes.

- Once the crusts have cooled slightly, take out the onions and divide them equally among the tart cases.

- Cut the brie into 12 even pieces and place them atop the onions. Sprinkle some herbs on them for garnish.

- Put the crusts back into the oven and bake them for about 15 minutes, until you notice the tops getting brown.

- As soon as they brown, take them out of the oven and serve.

- You can even keep the tartlets refrigerated and have them the next day.

Nutrition Information (per serving)

- Calories – 220 calories

- Fat – 12 grams

- Carbs – 2 grams

- Protein – 10 grams

Day 14

Low-Carb Veggie Fritters

These crispy delights are packed with some incredible nutrients. Typically, they are made using unsalted butter. However, as we would like to increase the fat content, we are going to make use of ghee. Whatever you choose, however, the result is delicious and crispy fritters.

Serving Size

12 fritters

Ingredients

4 medium eggs

1 zucchini, preferably large and grated

1 carrot, preferably medium and grated

½ celeriac, preferably medium and grated

1 cup sauerkraut (drained)

1 yellow onion, small and diced

½ teaspoon sea salt

½ teaspoon chili flakes, for flavor

2 tablespoons ghee or duck fat, for cooking

Instructions

- Pour water in a bowl. Add in the celeriac and carrots. Add the salt into the mixture. Stir and set it aside for about 15 minutes.

- Take another bowl and place a muslin cloth in it. Transfer your celeriac and carrots to the bowl.

- Add the zucchini and the sauerkraut.

- Next, squeeze out the water and any juices. Discard the liquid.

- Place the vegetables into a bowl once they are drained and mix them with eggs. Add your chili flakes for seasoning if you prefer.

- Place a pan over medium-low heat. Pour your ghee into the pan. Fry for about 5 or 6 minutes.

- Next, flip the fritters over and fry them on the other side for another 5 or 6 minutes.

- Repeat the process if needed until the fritters are cooked well.

Nutrition Information (per serving)

- Calories – 223 calories

- Fat – 11 grams

- Carbs – 5 grams

- Protein – 6 grams

We have reached halfway through your daily meal plan. At this point, you should be well acclimated to the new type of diet as you have already been incorporating it into your life for two weeks. You might not struggle with the diet as much as you did in the beginning.

Day 15 - 28

For the remaining days, you can simply combine what you have prepared during the first 14 days or repeat the diet all over again. One tip that you can follow is to start preparing your meals in the reverse order that you had prepared them for the first 14 days.

The choice is entirely yours.

24, 48, and 72-hour Fasts. Are They Even Possible?

Yes, they are.

Most people think of fasting for such long periods as completely crazy! How can you go 24 hours or more without food? And why would you do it?!

Many reasons.

Perhaps you might be traveling to another country and the airport or plane food might not suit your body (it is fairly common for many people). You might not want to resort to the plane food just because you are hungry. Oftentimes, it also depends on the plane you are traveling in. If you have chosen a low-budget airline, then you might not have complete faith in their food quality. Whatever your reasons are, you could use a 24-hour fast to make sure that you skip any unsuitable food until you reach a place where you can finally dig in to some good stuff.

In many cases, people might find the local food in the country they are visiting unsuitable for them. Let us suppose that you are traveling to Thailand for a business trip for about 48 hours. Let us also assume that Thai food and your stomach are not exactly BFFs. Instead of forcing yourself to eat the local food, you could fast until you are back home.

These are just some examples of why people would prefer to go fasting.

Of course, we cannot discount the most important factor: the cleansing of your body.

So how do you prepare yourself for each of the fasting periods mentioned above?

24 hour fast

The first thing that you should do is put your body into a state of ketosis. If you have been following our meal plan or if you have gotten started on it, then you have practically completed your initiation into ketosis.

On the morning of the day of the fast, drink a cup of water with a little sea salt added to it. This will replace the electrolytes in your body. It also helps lower cortisol levels which will help to reduce your stress. You see, you should aim to keep your stress levels low in the morning.

Additionally, make sure you get a good night's rest before you start the day of fasting. If you are sleep deprived, then your blood sugar levels increase and it enters into your kidneys. This causes you to urinate frequently, which in turn causes you to get thirsty really fast.

Once you have your water in the morning, you then have to wait for about two to three hours before you can consume coffee or tea, should you choose to. However, you need to make sure that you are having black coffee or plain tea only. No milk. No sugar.

During your fast, what you can also do, and which I recommend that you do, is drink mineral water. But make sure you do not drink too much of it as it could cause frequent urination.

What do you do if you do feel hungry? One of the important things to remember is that when you are in a state of ketosis you do not feel hungry because your body is deprived of essential nutrients. You feel hungry at specific times because your body has been trained to receive food during those times. In other words, your body is on autopilot and reacts to the circadian rhythm that you have set up for yourself. It is time for you to take back control of your appetite. To curb your hunger, you can drink coffee (black only). Coffee is one of the best appetite suppressants. It also promotes the production of ketone bodies in your body.

Do not consume artificial sweeteners. Despite what you hear about them, they are known to cause an insulin response in your body. Which is why it is preferable to stay away from them.

Make sure that you are also engaged in low-intensity exercises. These help you deplete liver glycogen, which eventually helps promote ketosis even more.

48 hour fast

A 48-hour fast might be difficult for beginners. I strongly recommend working on the 24-hour fast before you try out this fast. What you are doing here is trying to remain on a water diet for a 48-hour period. The primary purpose of this fast is to cleanse your body and give it an opportunity to heal. According to doctors who have looked into the water diet during a long fast, the water fast encourages rapid regeneration of the intestine's mucosal lining. This type of fasting also gives cells the ability to eliminate waste and rid the body of harmful toxins.

The best way to go about this type of fast is by getting into OMAD. Once you are comfortable around it, then you are ready to fast for a 48-hour period.

Let us assume that your last OMAD meal was at 7 pm. Your next course of action would be to head to bed and get a good night's sleep.

The next day, you are going to drink mineral water or water with sea salt in the morning to replenish your electrolytes.

During the afternoon, you can have your cup of coffee to reduce the feeling of hunger. For the rest of the day, you should drink mineral water frequently.

When you reach the evening, you might feel a pang of hunger. At this time, you simply have to take a glass of water and add one or two teaspoons of apple cider vinegar into it. ACV has practically zero calories. But what it also has is potassium and magnesium which replenishes the electrolytes in your body and help stave off hunger.

The first 24 hours of your fast is the most challenging time. Think of it like cresting a hill. The first 24 hours are like going uphill. You will feel the challenge. However, once you cross the top (the 24-hour mark), it is all a smooth downhill experience from there.

Finally, you should be having your final OMAD meal once you complete the fast.

72 hour fast

This is one of the most challenging fasts you will experience and I would highly recommend starting out with the 24-hour fast before you even think of venturing into the 72-hour fast.

Apart from that, there are a few protocols that you can follow before you begin your 72-hour fast.

The first being that you should be on your OMAD diet for at least three to five days. When you are on your OMAD diet, you are going to be significantly less hungry during the fasting period. Your body is going to produce ketones. It will cleanse itself of bad cells and proteins. It is starting to use good fats as its fuel source rather than carbs. In short, it will prepare you for the fast.

The second protocol that you should be following is loading your body with water and sodium. To find sodium in water, you should always opt for mineral water. As we saw before, your body tends to urinate when it has less sodium. Now, urinating itself is not a bad process. This is because you drop all those harmful substances that your body possesses. However, urination means that the water content in your body is slightly dipping. This means that you have to supplement the water lost during the process. Another question that you might ask is why sodium is vital to the body. The main reason is that sodium helps maintain the fluids in your body in a normal state, such as your body water. This means that you do not feel dehydrated quickly.

Another reason why sodium is important is that when your body has a lack of the substance, then you activate certain receptors in your body called NST receptors. These receptors send signals to your brain that you need to have food. More specifically, it craves foods with salt content, as salt contains high amounts of sodium. This means you start getting hungry really fast.

Once you have the above protocols set into place, you can practically ease your way into a long-term fast. It becomes easier and you do not feel the strong effects of hunger while you are fasting.

When you are fasting, make sure that you are consuming the below items only:

Water (mineral, tap or sparkling)

Coffee

Apple Cider Vinegar

Tea

When it comes to the kind of tea you are consuming, make sure you take in only green tea. This is because green tea has epigallocatechin gallate, or EGCG. One of the most important functions of the EGCG is that it helps our body activate certain enzymes and genetic processes that help us during our fast. You feel more in control of your appetite.

Another important component of green tea is theanine. This important ingredient of tea helps your body produce more gamma-aminobutyric acid. This acid helps you remain calmer and satiate you during your fast.

Why is remaining calm essential? Any time you get anxious, stressed, or experience negative mental states, your body releases higher amounts of cortisol. This hormone increases the insulin levels in your body. Your sugar levels then drop and you eventually become hungry.

Finally, get plenty of rest. Do not skip out on a good night's sleep. You do not want to stress your body, either physically or mentally.

With these tips in mind, you are ready to begin an incredible and rejuvenating fasting experience.

Chapter 8: Keto Autophagy Lifestyle

You have now entered the OMAD lifestyle. It has its ups and downs, but you are finding yourself able to manage your fast so far. You feel confident about the fast and of your capability to deal with it.

Is there anything else that you need to consider?

There is.

You see, getting used to the fast is just one side of the coin, you need to maintain the lifestyle as well.

Here are a few tips to enjoy a comfortable and rewarding keto autophagy experience.

Stay Hydrated

This is a no brainer. We have already seen how hydration helps with your fast. You need to ensure that you refill your body's water levels. As your kidneys produce urine, you expunge your body of harmful materials. That in itself is not a bad thing. Urinating is one of the ways your body gets rid of waste. However, when you urinate, your body water levels become irregular and you can lower the levels of water and sodium in your body. This means that you need to replenish the water levels of your body.

Eat Your Meals Slowly

This is different from chewing your food many times. Often, people tend to gobble down their food quickly. When you eat slowly, you help your body digest food more effectively. You also lose weight more quickly and without much discomfort. At the same time, you feel satiated with each meal you have. What you are doing by eating slowly is that you are giving your body the time to extract the nutrients from each bite you take. That means you feel more satisfied with your meal.

When you eat fast, you tend to push down your portion. Which is why many people still feel hungry even after having a rather fulfilling meal. If you rush through your food you affect your digestion. Your meals become a stressful situation. Your body might send signals indicating that the meal was over too soon and it probably means that you did not have enough. Add to that the fact that sometimes the stress your body endures gets translated to a rise in cortisol. We do not want that happening.

Improve Your Sleep Patterns

If you are not having proper sleep, then your body will automatically elevate its levels of stress hormones. This leads to irregular blood sugar levels. I recommend that you head to bed before 11 pm. Ensure that you are sleeping in a dark room. Keep mobile phones and other devices away from you as radiation from these devices can affect your sleep. Make sure you are not using these devices for at least an hour before you sleep. I also recommend getting 7 to 9 hours of good sleep each night.

How to Adapt to OMAD

Societal Pressure

Just take a look around you. There is no shortage of foods available. There are stores at nearly every corner of your area. You have vending machines providing you quick snacks. Your refrigerator, kitchen, and probably even your room might be filled with options that could tempt you out of a keto diet.

However, these temptations can be managed.

What you might find difficult to manage is the pressure you receive from society. You see, most people are not used to taking up a keto diet. It becomes rather difficult for them or they give up too easily. Others simply choose to not believe in the diet, thinking that it is simply an absurd idea concocted by someone to make a lot of money.

But the reality is that in today's world, people are becoming more aware. They want to focus on something that is backed by science, practice, and results. When the keto diet entered the scene, there were a lot of skeptics. Is this another way to bamboozle us out of our money? Am I going to do something that does not generate any result?

Over time, science decided to jump in on the subject of keto dieting. Scientists and society wanted to know whether the diet actually works. As more and more facts began to pile up, researchers realized that the keto diet is not based on a random collection of facts.

It is a scientifically studied method.

But even so, you might feel compelled to shift away from the diet because the people around you might convince you to do so. Or you might look at others enjoying all the meals in the world and it might make you wonder if it's worth taking on the keto diet.

Let me tell you that people have found results through ketogenic autophagy and OMAD routines.

I am not just referring to physical changes. I am talking about improving your focus, attention, memory, and productivity. I am talking about longevity. Because keto does not simply throw in a process for the sake of doing so. A keto diet focuses on certain aspects of our life and chooses to enhance those areas.

So do not worry about what others say. You are on a path to bring a healthy change into your life. And while it may be a difficult path (when is progress not difficult?) there is a big reward at the end of the journey.

Hunger Levels

You are going to feel the discomfort of hunger when you begin your OMAD journey. After all, you are plunging yourself into a new lifestyle after decades of sticking to specific routines, patterns, and indulgences.

It takes time to adjust.

However, there are many ways you can deal with hunger while you are on your OMAD diet. I have already shown you steps to work on your hunger while you are in the middle of a 24, 48, or 72-hour diet. You can apply the same steps to manage hunger during OMAD.

Remember that the key to a successful one meal a day plan lies in your willpower. Sure, it is challenging to go through a diet plan. However, the challenge becomes manageable when you realize that your body is not the one demanding food, your brain is.

Your body has all the nutrients it requires. Unfortunately, your brain is used to decades of conditioning and is refusing to let go of its old belief systems and habits.

When you master your mind, you can master your body.

That notion becomes true when you are going through OMAD.

Breaking Fast: How to Break Fast the Right Way

When you are ready to break your fast your body is primed to take in the nutrients that you provide. It's like a vacuum, switch it on and whoosh! In goes your food faster than you can spell the word "digest".

This means that it is ready to absorb all those nutrients quickly. While you may think that your stomach working really fast means that you get more nutrients into your body, then that is not true. Remember our section on eating slowly? There is a reason we included that. We are aiming for your digestive processes to take in all the nutrients without sending any of them to the waste bin.

In a similar way, do not break your fast by eating something.

Get your body ready. Let it know that there is awesome stuff incoming.

To get your body into a state of readiness, try the below techniques:

Drink ACV, Lemon Water, or Bone Broth

We had already established that ACV is not just vital for your body during fasting but it also helps you gain some extra elements vital for you.

Lemon water is known to improve digestion. This is why having it before your meal preps your body to work on your food more effectively.

Similarly, bone broth plays a vital role in promoting digestive health.

There really is no better or worse option. Simply choose the drink that you prefer and have it before you begin to break your fast.

For Muslims, the month of Ramadan is a holy month. It involves the process of fasting from dawn till dusk as part of their mandatory ritual. Ramadan occurs every year and Muslims prepare their body for the fast in many ways.

What is important to note is the routine they follow during the fasting process. You see, when it comes time to break their fast, they do not immediately sit down to eat. They most commonly consume dates and follow that with a glass of water.

They are preparing their body for receiving food.

Of course, we are not going to eat dates because the fruit has high sugar content.

However, the concept of breaking your fast by preparing your body in advance is still a vital component of Muslim fasting.

What we are doing is fairly similar, minus all the high carb and high sugar foods.

To successfully break your fast, make sure you take in a glass of water with two teaspoons of ACV, a glass of lemon water, or bone broth 30 minutes to around 1 hour before you plan to eat a solid meal.

Supplementary Support

Taking supplements can help you with your fasting. They not only help you manage your hunger, but they infuse your body with essential nutrients. Let us examine some of the supplements that you can take during OMAD and the kind of benefits they provide your body.

Vitamin D3

If you would like your body to absorb more calcium and improve the growth of your bones, then you need vitamin D3. When you have little of the substance in your body, your bones could turn fragile or, in some cases, misshapen. Adding a little vitamin D during your fast helps you sustain yourself better during the fast.

Vitamin D plays an important role in the maintenance of calcium and phosphorus levels in the blood. These two compounds influence the way your bones develop tremendously.

Additionally, we also need vitamin D to absorb calcium in the intestines and to ensure that too much calcium does not get excreted through the kidneys.

Fish Oil

In the past decade, many health physicians and doctors have recommended fish oil to their patients. But what makes this supplement so popular?

For one, fish oil contains omega-3 fatty acids. These are helpful for the following reasons:

- Reduce blood pressure

- Lower the instances of your heart picking up an abnormal rhythm

- Lower the chances of strokes and heart attacks

Fish oil becomes especially important when you are working out. Combine all of the above benefits and the fact that fish oil reduces muscle soreness and joint pains, then you have the ideal supplement to take for your workouts.

L-Carnitine

L-Carnitine is an amino acid that is naturally produced in your body. As you grow older, your body reduces the supply of L-Carnitine. This causes your body to slow down, have reduced energy, and prevents you from enjoying an active lifestyle. As your activity reduces, you easily gain weight.

When you are fasting, you should aim to be as active as possible. In order to help you with that, you can take L-Carnitine as a supplement. The amino acid becomes especially useful when you are about to workout, giving you a quick boost of energy for your exercises.

Do note that the best time to take the supplement would be first thing in the morning and on an empty stomach. You could also take it later during the day, but make sure you are taking it at least 30 minutes before you break your fast.

Turmeric

Turmeric is a popular spice in India. In fact, many of the dishes in the country include turmeric as a vital ingredient. If you've ever wondered how Indian curries gain their yellow color, then you now know the answer why. Yes indeed, it is turmeric.

Indians consider turmeric as having medicinal properties.

In wasn't until recently that science has started to understand why Indians believe that turmeric provides them with health benefits. One of the most important components of turmeric is curcumin. Why is this component vital? Curcumin is what gives turmeric its anti-inflammatory properties. It is also a strong anti-oxidant. Which is why, you can choose to add turmeric either into your food, or you can have supplements made out of turmeric. Either way, you are making sure that your body receives the right amount of curcumin.

Exercising During Fasting

When you exercise during your OMAD diet, you are forcing your body to remove fat. This is because the process of burning fats in your body is managed by your sympathetic nervous system (SNS). Why is this important? Well, one of the major ways in which you can activate your SNS is by exercising and lack of food.

This is why numerous health and fitness experts recommend including exercises as part of your fasting regime. As we saw before, resistance training can be incorporated into your diet.

Remember the following tips before you start performing your exercises and while you are exercising:

Always warm up before you dive into any exercise.

Stick to a routine that is comfortable for you. Do not overdo it.

Focus on using the right form and posture. Do not think about momentum. You might have noticed people in the gym using momentum and showing how they are exerting a lot of energy. This is not always because they are working really hard. Sometimes, it is because they are performing the wrong posture and that tends to force people to add more energy than is necessary.

Chapter 9: What to Do if Your Weight Loss Plateaus

You have now been following a strict diet. You have been working hard to maintain a healthy OMAD diet and improve your exercise routines. You can see progress. Your reward for exercising has been seeing your weight go down and your overall health improve. All of a sudden and for no reason you can understand, the weight on the scale has stopped decreasing. What the heck?! Did you do something wrong?! Has the diet stopped working?

Fear not, my friend. You have only reached a point that every individual who goes on a diet reaches. You have reached a weight-loss plateau.

Do not feel disheartened. There is nothing to worry about. It is completely normal for weight loss to slow down a bit and sometimes even just remain at a particular point for a while.

When you begin to understand the mechanisms behind a weight-loss plateau, you have the power to know how to react and prevent giving up on your OMAD diet.

During the initial period of your weight-loss regime, you might notice a rapid drop in your weight. You might feel a sense of exhilaration.

This drop happens because when you curb down your calories, your body gets the necessary energy by releasing its reserves of glycogen. Glycogen is a type of carbohydrate that is found in the liver and the muscles.

Glycogen contains water. This is why, when glycogen is used by the body for energy, it releases water. This water release causes your weight to plummet down like a skydiver in freefall.

When you see the rapid drop in weight, it is definitely a wonderful moment. However, it is a temporary situation.

As you continue to lose weight, you also some muscles as well. Here is the thing about muscles, they help you maintain the rate at which calories are burnt in your body. In other words, they manage the speed of your metabolism. This is why, the more weight you lose, the more muscles are lost. This causes your metabolism to lower, leading to a decrease in the rate of burning calories. Eventually, the rate at which you lose weight declines.

At this point, your metabolism has slowed down. But it does not stop entirely. This is why you are still losing weight, just not at the same rate as before. Eventually, you reach a point where you are consuming the same amount of calories as you burn.

That is when your weight loss plateaus.

Additionally, because our bodies have ways to increase our resilience and longevity during times of fasting, our brains will trigger a variety of mechanisms to keep us from losing more weight. Why does this happen?

Evolution.

Back when our ancestors were hunting for food, they often faced situations of famine. They had no technology to protect them during those times and starvation was a common problem. In fact, some of the mass exoduses in human history were made to avoid famine and find better places for food. But I digress. Back to our bodies.

As time went on, our bodies evolved to protect us during times of famine. It did not want us to lose more weight because weight loss meant getting weaker. And if people got weaker, then that meant they were next in line to be on the buffet menu of a saber-tooth tiger.

No one likes to be on the menu of a saber-tooth tiger.

Nowadays, there are no sabretooth tigers. But that does not mean that our evolutionary traits have been expunged from our bodies. They still exist.

So when you enter a state of fasting, your brain thinks it is experiencing famine. That's when it activates mechanisms to prevent weight loss.

As you can see, nothing to worry about. Not even saber-tooth tigers.

To begin losing weight, all you need to do is either have more physical activity on a daily basis or reduce the calories you eat. Thankfully for us, OMAD means you increase activities and decrease calories. You are getting the best of both worlds. When you use the same level of physical activity that you had before you began your diet, then you may not lose too much weight.

Track Your Calories. Recalculate Your Macros.

To count or not to count, that is an interesting question. When you are losing calories, you might feel conflicted about measuring your calories. On one hand, you may not want to see how your progress is going on. Will you be surprised? Will you be disappointed? Questions like that make you hesitant about checking your calories. When you maintain a record or keep a track of the calories you consume from your meals, you encourage yourself to make better choices. You become responsible for the changes happening to your body. You are now accountable for the results that occur because of your dieting. Moreover, you can keep a constant check on your progress.

You can use this online tool to calculate your macros https://www.active.com/fitness/calculators/bmr

Whether you receive good news or bad news, you should have a sense of awareness about what is happening to your body. Do not fool yourself into thinking that something is happening. Be certain. Be informed. You see, you cannot fool yourself with arbitrary numbers and statistics when you jot down your calorie count. Recording your food consumption and knowing what you eat is an important part of losing weight. It is better to eat a wonderful salad than to waste time-consuming a nutritious meal that may not even be working out for you.

Your choices matter. Make informed ones.

This is why your decisions matter when you realize that your weight plateaus. Imagine working so hard but not realizing that nothing is happening to your body. Never put yourself in that situation. Measure your calories and recalculate your macros so that when your weight loss plateaus, you know what to do next.

Increase Protein Intake. Increase Exercise Frequency.

Protein is good. Do not let anyone convince you otherwise. Of course, you need to maintain it within a moderate level. However, when you begin to notice your weight loss slowing down, then it is time to increase your intake of proteins. One of the best parts of the recipes mentioned in this book is that they are chock full of protein. So any time you want to have more protein, simply increase the serving sizes or portions of the food.

Moreover, make sure that you increase the amount you exercise.

Why is working out more important? Well, you are now consuming the same amount of calories that you burn. At this point, you need to burn more calories so that you can encourage weight loss.

And that is where exercises become important. You burn an incredible amount of calories through exercises. This resets the balance and you start seeing the weighing scale show progress.

Furthermore, do you remember when we talked about how you begin to lose muscles during fasting? Guess how you can reverse that and reduce the amount of muscles that you have lost?

Yep, exercise.

So make sure you have a balanced workout plan along with your fasting routine so that you can gain as many benefits as possible from your OMAD diet.

Fat Fast

There is another technique that you can use to get out of the plateau phase: a fat fast.

What exactly is a fat fast?

You know what a water fast entails. You are basically consuming mainly liquids so that you can fast for a long period of time. The long-period fasting where you fast from 24 to 72 hours is a type of water fast.

In a similar way, a fat fast is where you consume only or mainly fats. In a fat fast, you should aim to receive about 80% to 90% of your calories from fat. The remaining calories can be received from protein.

When you are engaged in a fat fast, you are recommended to have around 1,000–1,200 calories per day.

If you analyze a fat fast, then you realize that it is not actually a fast. What you are doing is ramping the amount of fats you consume and decreasing most of the other components of food. A fat fast imitates the biological properties of avoiding too much food by placing your body into a state of ketosis. When your body hits the ketosis stage, then you begin to use fats. You lower dependency on carbs.

A fat fast is specifically created to induce a calorie deficit in your body. Such a deficit is vital for your weight. A fat fast also depletes the body's reserves of carbs so that you are pushed into a state of ketosis and begin burning more fat.

If you would like to adopt a fat fast technique into your diet, then you have to ensure you boost foods that give you healthy fats and maintain such a diet for at least 3 days.

When you notice that your weight loss has gained momentum again, then you can return to your regular keto diet and continue maintaining your keto routines.

But there are a few things you must know about a fat fast.

You see, some people think that a fat fast is a quick way to enter ketosis, it could very well become an important component of their diet.

That is not a good move.

You see, fat fasting does not provide the necessary amount of protein, calories and various other micronutrients that are important for your health. This is why it is not a long-term solution for weight loss or a diet plan in and of itself. I ask you to exercise caution if you are extending a fat fast for long periods.

Apart from that one caveat, fat fasting is healthy in the short-term. It is designed for a specific purpose: accelerating your weight loss process. You should only use it for that specific purpose.

However, I have given you loads of options for recipes. So which ones should you eat to make the best use of your fat fast?

Use dishes that contain bacon, salmon, eggs, olive oil, mayonnaise, zucchini, butter (even if it is unsalted), and nuts. There are numerous dishes you can prepare that contain the above ingredients. In many of the dishes, you can find a combination of the above ingredients. Additionally, include coffee and tea as your liquid option during your fat fast.

With that, you are ready to get back on the road to weight loss!

Conclusion

You have started your OMAD diet.

You are ready to make the most out of it.

You are now on your third or fourth day and everything is going good.

All of a sudden, you are invited to a social event. It could be someone's birthday party or a meeting between friends. You decide to attend the event. Soon, you find out that your friends or family are about to indulge in a nice juicy steak and they are hoping you join them. But that would mean you are going to have a second meal!

Gosh!

The nightmare!

Perhaps it is time to disappoint your friends or family and let them know that you won't be having that steak no matter what.

First of all, relax.

You see, this is a common problem among many people who undertake OMAD, they feel that they have to be strict about what they eat at all times.

That is not true at all.

Of course, you shouldn't indulge yourself every opportunity you get else you are defeating the purpose of an OMAD diet.

However, when it comes to social occasions, it is alright to loosen up a bit and enjoy the moment. It is not the end of the world.

When you have certain obligations, then you can go ahead and indulge yourself a bit. What you should pay attention to is the idea that you are not overindulging yourself or eating too much frequently.

You are allowed to have a second meal once in a while when the occasion calls for it. Remember that this does not mean you get to have cheat days. Rather, you might have to be part of certain social obligations. You don't want to be seen as the person who just dampened the mood of everyone at the party.

So relax and have your second meal. Just make sure that you are back on your diet the next day.

But having a second meal is just one of the concerns people have about their OMAD plan. Sometimes, it boils down to asking oneself just how many days in a week should one keep an OMAD diet. I have known people to become so obsessed with their diet that they maintain it seven days a week and then find themselves facing a serious withdrawal problem.

I am not saying that you should not keep an OMAD diet seven days a week. Rather, what you should be looking at are your goals.

What are you aiming to achieve?

If you would like to encourage a better lifestyle for yourself, then you could consider keeping an OMAD diet for 5 days a week. You will receive enough benefits during that phase to make sure that you cleanse your body, rejuvenate your cells and proteins, and find more physical and mental stability in your life.

It is true that you cannot simply indulge in high carb food during the days that you are not on your OMAD diet. You cannot have delicious and healthy salads for five days and then head over to McDonald's and pop two cheeseburgers with extra patties with a side of extra-large fries and coke on the sixth day!

You are making changes in your life and you have to maintain that change.

However, you can deviate from your OMAD diet on the sixth and seventh day. You can choose to have a nice breakfast after your 5-day OMAD plan. Perhaps even have a light lunch. And then get back to your OMAD diet again the following week.

Do note that this process has proven to be challenging for some people as they end up being reluctant to go back to their OMAD diet.

But the fact remains; you can have cheat days in your OMAD diet. The only difference is that during your cheat days, you are still eating good food. You are just having a little extra portion of it.

Remember this, you can always enjoy a delicious meal without having to resort to junk. There are plenty of food options where you might be adding a bit more carbs than usual but you are not overdosing on them.

OMAD is meant to add numerous benefits into your life. You have to enter it using a plan. When you plan out your approach, you know exactly what you would like to take from the diet.

If you are aiming to lose weight, then you know how much effort you are going to place in the OMAD process. You are not tricking yourself into thinking that things are going to be easy.

In the same way, if you are planning to maintain a healthy lifestyle then you might go a little easy on yourself. This will prevent you from thinking that OMAD is a rather scary diet to be part of.

Do note this: cheat days are going to happen.

You are going to have one of those days you cannot avoid.

My recommendation is don't avoid those days.

Enjoy yourself and live in the moment. Because you know that once you are done, you are going to get back to your diet anyway. You know that you are not straying too far from your routines and that your main goal will always be to keep a balanced and healthy diet routine.

Enjoy the process and know that you are not adopting OMAD into your life because it is just another cool fad. You are using it to better yourself.

You are creating a change that will have lasting impressions on both your physical and mental health. In fact, because one of the main components of OMAD is to maintain your stress levels, you are going to learn how to manage stress, prevent negative emotions and mental states from taking over your mind, and keep a calm demeanor. In many ways, you are becoming a master of not just your body, but your mind as well.

Progress always involves a bit of hard work. But that fact should not concern you. Rather, it should help you realize that you are an individual capable of making some incredible changes in your life.

With that, I hope you enjoy the journey you take for your OMAD diet. I sincerely hope for your success and that you find the results you seek. After all, you only get one life.

Keep it going long.

Keto Diet on the Go

Your Guide to Low-Carb Friendly Options at America's Favorite Restaurants

Written By

Jason Michaels

Introduction

You've conquered the first step by getting your body into ketosis. One of the many perks of this eating lifestyle is its sustainability. There are so many good foods that you can eat while in ketosis that will keep you satisfied and you won't even miss the bread! However, it's one thing to stick to the plan when you're doing your own meal prep. It's a whole new ballgame when you take your new eating habits out into the world. There are a few things you can do before reaching the restaurant of choice that will hopefully make the process a bit easier.

First, when possible, try not go out to eat on an empty stomach. If you're already somewhat satisfied you'll be able to resist temptations that much better. Even if you chug a glass of room temperature water before you leave, your stomach will feel more full.

If you've planned ahead, do your research before getting to the restaurant. Almost every chain restaurant has its full menu publically available. Decide which direction you want to take your meal and any off-menu modifications you might want to make. That way, when it comes time to order you'll know exactly what you want and how many carbs it will cost you.

Pack food ahead of time for trips. That will make you less likely to splurge on carby snacks at the gas station or airport.

Finally, don't stress out! It's understandable that asking for off-menu items can be a bit intimidating. There is always the risk that your dining companion might not understand or the order might arrive incorrect or incomplete. And that's okay! Because it will happen, on occasion, but at the end of the day, you are the one that matters.

So get ready to dive into the low-carb faction of the restaurant world. Bon appetit!

Side Note: net carbs are calculated by subtracting total fiber from total carbs

There are plenty of books on this subject on the market, thanks again for choosing this one! Every effort was made to ensure it is full of as much useful information as possible, please enjoy!

Chapter 1: Keto Options: Well-Known Chain Restaurants

Eating out, in general, can make it difficult to maintain dieting goals. Sticking to a diet at our favorite, well-known restaurants can up the challenge considerably. Thankfully, healthier trends in food preparation and low-carb options made available have made an appearance in a wide variety of our better-known chains.

Denny's

Good ol' Denny's; comforting, easy on the pocketbook, and they're always open! Resisting favorites could be difficult at this family favorite sit-down restaurant, but where there is a will, there is a way. And thankfully, there are quite a few ways to make these potentially carb-loaded meals much more keto friendly. Many of these low-carb options are appropriate for breakfast, lunch, or dinner.

T-Bone Steak & Eggs: This is about as perfect for low-carb eating as you can get...if all you were served was the steak and the eggs. Forgoing sides is a sacrifice that must be made, so to keep this favorite keto friendly, leave out extras such as toast and hash browns and it comes to about 1g net carbs.

Grand Slam (build-your-own): The Grand Slam is definitely on the favorites list. Here is a list of ingredients you could use to customize it to your liking and diet goals:

Bacon (2 strips= 1g net carbs), turkey bacon (2 strips= 1g net carbs), sausage (2 links= 0g net carbs), eggs (2= 1g net carbs), egg whites (2= 1g net carbs), grilled ham (3oz. slice= 3g net carbs), gouda-apple chicken sausage (1 link= 2g net carbs).

Use this list to mix and match to your liking, staying away from the pancakes, of course.

Favorite Omelettes: Denny's offers a variety of omelettes that are typically Keto friendly as they are, just be sure to leave out the "carby" sides:

Ham & Cheese Omelette: 7g net carbs

Ultimate Omelette®: 8g net carbs

Loaded Veggie Omelette: 7g net carbs

Philly Cheese-steak Omelette: 11g net carbs

Skillets: Denny's skillets are another great option, just be sure to get them without the potatoes. There was no data available on the exact net carbs on the skillets, but as long as they are potato free they should all fall below 10g:

Fit Fare® Veggie Skillet

Crazy Spicy Skillet (option to add eggs)

Supreme Skillet (option to add eggs)

Wild Alaska Salmon Skillet

Santa Fe Skillet (option to add eggs)

Salads & Sides: You can never go wrong with a salad! Well, I guess technically you can, but as long as you stick to these low-carb options you'll be on the right track:

Prime Rib Cobb Salad (no dressing): 12g net carbs

Veggies with Ranch Dip: 3g net carbs

Avocado Chicken Caesar Salad (16 oz.): 8g net carbs

Tilapia Ranchero (no bread): 3g net carbs

T-Bone Steak (no bread): 5g net carbs

Sirloin Steak (no bread): 3g net carbs

Burgers/Sandwiches: None of these options will start as low-carb because of the bread and some of the condiments. To make these sandwiches keto friendly, order without the bread, possibly in a lettuce wrap, avoid sugary condiments such as BBQ sauce and ketchup, and skip the fries or substitute with cut veggies. Try to limit or avoid fruit as sides.

Condiments: Condiment options will probably be very similar across the board at any restaurant, but here are some specific to Denny's:

Ranch Dressing (1.5oz): 1g net carbs

Buffalo Sauce (2oz): 2g net carbs

Blue Cheese Dressing (1.5oz): 3g net carbs

Caesar Dressing (1.5oz): 0g net carbs

Italian Dressing (Fat free, 1.5oz): 4g net carbs

Sour Cream (1.5oz): 2g net carbs

IHOP

IHOP options will be very similar to Denny's and the same rules for entrees, sandwiches and burgers will apply: skip the bread, potatoes, and sweet condiments. Some of the main menu, however, can be ordered with little to no alterations.

Omelettes: Something to keep in mind; some of the research has discovered that IHOP puts pancake batter in their eggs when they make the omelettes, which obviously has an effect on the net carbs. Be sure to request real eggs when ordering.

Colorado Omelette: 13g net carbs

Avocado, Bacon, Cheese Omelette: 5g net carbs

Corned Beef Hash & Cheese Omelette: 20g net carbs

Bacon Temptation Omelette: 10g net carbs

Bacon, Sausage, and Eggs: When in doubt, keep it simple...good ol' bacon and eggs! Eggs (basic serving size is usually 2) can be fried, poached, scrambled, or boiled and they will contain about 1-2g net carbs. Sausage or bacon are usually about 1g net carbs for an order. Order just bacon and/or sausage and eggs (no sides) and you'll have a fulfilling meal that will keep you in ketosis.

Salads/Dressings: As with any salad, the danger is most often in the dressing, both the type and the quantity.

Grilled Chicken Cobb: 10g net carbs (without the dressing)

House Salad: 3g net carbs (without the dressing)

Caesar Salad (side, 12g net carbs, without the dressing)

The dressings are what launch the net carbs upward, so take care when ordering! Get the dressing on the side to help keep the carb load down.

Waffle House

Yet another diner style, comforting, carb-laden restaurant. And still, there are plenty of low carb options to choose from.

Omelettes: Avoid sides (toast, hash browns, etc.).

Ham & Cheese Omelette: 10g net carbs

Fiesta Omelette: 7g net carbs

Cheese-steak Omelette: 6g net carbs

Breakfast Staples

Bacon (3 slices): 0g net carbs

Country Ham (1 slice): 0g net carbs

Sausage (2 patties): 0g net carbs

Eggs w/ Cheese (2 eggs, equivalent of 1 slice of cheese): 1g net carbs

Sausage Egg & Cheese Wrap: 25g Net Carbs

Meat: Most meat choices, without any kind of sauce or gravy, are going to be 0g net carbs.

Burgers/Sandwiches: Same rule applies as before; skip the bread, sweet condiments, and fries. Maybe try adding a fried egg on top of a bunless burger to make it more interesting.

California Pizza Kitchen

In order to stay low carb at California Pizza Kitchen, you may have to forgo the pizza. However, their low carb options are still very good and will provide a fulfilling meal while remaining in ketosis.

Salads

Italian Chopped Salad (half portion): 9g net carbs

Classic Caesar Salad (full portion): 12g net carbs

Roasted Veggie & Grilled Shrimp Salad (half portion): 17g net carbs

California Cobb Salad (full portion, including ranch dressing): 13g net carbs

Appetizers/Entrees

Lettuce Wraps (order with chicken or shrimp or both!)

Grilled Chicken Chimichurri: 13g net carbs

Fire-Roasted Chile Relleno: 20g net carbs

Grilled Chicken Breast (no sauces/sides): 0g net carbs

Power Bowls: These are definitely healthier options; for keto diets, they may still need to be tweaked just a bit. No net carb info available, but here are some suggestions to make sure these bowls stay keto friendly:

Shanghai Power Bowl: This meal comes with shrimp and a variety of vegetables such as cauliflower, baby broccoli, carrots, and zucchini. It also includes Forbidden Rice® and house made Shanghai sauce, both of which should probably be held off (or at least on the side) to keep the carbs down.

Santa Fe Bowl: This bowl includes lime chicken, sweet corn, tomatoes, black beans, avocado, poblano peppers, red cabbage, and toasted pepitas on top of spinach and cilantro farro. It is served with CPK's house made ranch. To keep this bowl keto friendly, it would be best to skip the corn and ask for dressing on the side.

Banh Mi Bowl: This bowl consists of baby kale, quinoa, mint, and cilantro topped by grilled chicken, radishes, watermelon, avocado, carrots, bean sprouts, cucumbers, scallions, and sesame seeds. It comes with CPK's chili and lime vinaigrette and Serrano peppers. While quinoa is very healthy, it is also very high in protein. Unused protein is broken down into sugar and stored as fat.

Cauliflower Crust: CPK has recently come out with a cauliflower crust, reportedly consisting of cauliflower, rice flour, mozzarella, and some spices and herbs. This is great news for vegetarians but perhaps not so much for keto and low-carb as one slice is 90 calories and has 14g net carbs. It might be best to stick with non-pizza meals in order to remain in ketosis.

Chili's

Chili's actually has a section in their menu called "Guiltless Grills". Some items on this part of the menu may be a bit too high in starch, which bumps net carbs up to 50g and over. However, there are a few specific dishes that are perfect for the keto diet (all listed not including the sides that come with some of the entrees).

Guiltless Grills & Other Main Dishes

Guiltless Cedar Plank Tilapia: Seasoned tilapia fillet with Chili's house made pico de gallo and served on a cedar plank; 3g net carbs.

Guiltless Grilled Salmon: 8oz of salmon seasoned and seared; 5g net carbs.

Salmon with Garlic and Herbs: 1g net carbs

Guiltless Carne Asada Steak Sirloin: The meat is seasoned and flame grilled and also comes with the house made pico de gallo; 5g net carbs.

Spicy Garlic & Lime Grilled Shrimp: 7g net carbs

Pepper Pals Grilled Chicken Platter (on the kids' menu): 4g net carbs

Chili's Classic Sirloins: 1g net carbs

Starters

Caesar Salad (side portion, no croutons!): approximately 6g net carbs

Jason Michaels & Thomas Hawthorn

Triple Dipper Wings over Buffalo with Blue Cheese: 2g net carbs

Cup Chicken Enchilada: 8g net carbs

Terlinga Chili (cup): 7g net carbs

Lunch Combo House Salad (Hold the dressing): 9g net carbs

Extras/Sides

Dressings: Blue Cheese, Avocado Ranch, and Caesar

Avocado Slices

Side of Guacamole (small)

Sautéed Mushrooms

All Cheeses

Sour Cream

Steamed Broccoli

Cut veggies (celery, carrots)

Applebee's

Applebee's also has a low carb section on their menu, making it much easier to pick keto friendly meals.

Starters

Double Crunch Bone-In Wings (either with blue cheese or ranch dressing): 13g net carbs

Double Crunch Bone-In Wings (no sauce or dressing): 10g net carbs

Double Crunch Bone-In Wings (classic Buffalo): 13g net carbs

Main Dishes (from the grill)

Doubled-Glazed Baby Back Ribs (both half rack and full rack, no sauce): 0g net carbs

Fire-Grilled Shrimp Skewer: 1g net carbs

12oz Top Sirloin (Butcher's Reserve): 0g net carbs

USDA Top Sirloin 6oz: 1g net carbs

USDA Top Sirloin 8oz: 2g net carbs

Jason Michaels & Thomas Hawthorn

Shrimp 'N Parmesan Sirloin: 5g net carbs

Grilled Chicken Breast: 0g net carbs

Lunch Dishes

Thai Shrimp Salad: 12g net carbs

Tomato Basil Soup (cup): 13g net carbs

Southwest Black Bean Soup (cup): 12g net carbs

Grilled Chicken Caesar Salad (no croutons!): 8g net carbs

House Salads: Some of these salads are a bit higher in the carb range than you might want, especially if you plan on getting an entrée as well. Be mindful of dressing choice/quantity and leave off extras such as croutons, chips, fruit, and nuts.

House Salad w/ Buttermilk Ranch: 13g net carbs

House Salad w/ Garlic Caesar: 13g net carbs

House Salad w/ Blue Cheese: 13g net carbs

House Salad w/ Lemon Olive Oil Vinaigrette: 10g net carbs

House Salad w/ Mexi Ranch: 13g net carbs

House Salad w/ Italian: 15g net carbs

House Salad w/ Green Goddess: 12g net carbs

Small Caesar: 9g net carbs

Green Goddess Wedge Salad: 9g net carbs

House Salad (no dressing): 10g net carbs

Sides

Garlicky Green Beans w/ Bacon: 7g net carbs

Fire-Grilled Veggies: 6g net carbs

Steamed Broccoli: 3g net carbs

Wendy's

As with other restaurants serving burger and sandwiches, all of these low-carb options from Wendy's are bunless.

Jason Michaels *&* Thomas Hawthorn

Burger & Meat Options (no condiments or toppings)

Jr. Hamburger Patty: 0g net carbs

Single Hamburger Patty: 0g net carbs

Grilled Chicken Breast: 3g net carbs

Applewood Smoked Bacon (1 strip): 0g net carbs

Toppings/Condiments: The stand-alone meat options are very low in net carbs. Which means you can add to your order as you keep track of the carb count in these condiments and toppings.

Cheeses: American 1 slice= 1g net carbs, Asiago 1 slice= 1g net carbs, cheddar 1 slice= 0g net carbs, shredded cheddar= 1g net carbs, cheddar cheese sauce= 1g net carbs

Mayonnaise: 0g net carbs

Mustard: 0g net carbs

Pickles, onions, and iceberg lettuce: all 0g net carbs

Tomato: 1 slice= 1g net carbs

Tartar Sauce: 0g net carbs

Salads

Garden Salad (without dressing and croutons): 5g net carbs

Caesar Salad (without dressing and croutons): 4g net carbs

Sauces/Dressing

Ranch: 2g net carbs

Buttermilk Ranch (dipping sauce): 2g net carbs

Light Ranch: 2g net carbs

Italian: 4g net carbs

Lemon Garlic Caesar: 2g net carbs

Thousand Island: 5g net carbs

Meal Pairing Ideas: Now that we know individual options, we can mix and match meals. These won't necessarily have a spot on the actual menu, but they do fulfill the requirements for low-carb options.

Three Double-Stack Cheeseburgers (dry, no bun) with pickles, wrapped in lettuce: 3g net carbs

Grilled Chicken (dry, no bun), garden side salad w/ ranch, Diet Coke: 7g net carbs

Two Jr. Bacon Cheeseburgers (dry, no bun) with Caesar salad (no dressing or croutons), and small Minute Maid Lemonade: 11g net carbs

Triple Baconator (dry, no bun) mayo on the side, bottle of water: 3g net carbs

KFC

Everything about KFC says "comfort food". There is nothing specifically on the menu labeled as low-carb, but if KFC is absolutely the last option for a meal, there is a smart way to order to stay on the keto diet.

Meal Ideas

There aren't a lot of chicken options that will stick with the keto diet, so the Kentucky Grilled Chicken Breast is probably the only way to go:

Two Kentucky Grilled Chicken Breasts with a small side of green beans and maybe a side of creamy buffalo dip comes to about 6g net carbs.

Sides

Caesar Salad (no dressing): 1g net carbs

Side Salad (no dressing): 1g net carbs

Sauce

Creamy Buffalo: 2g net carbs

Buttermilk Ranch: 2g net carbs

Dressing

Marzetti Light Italian: 2g net carbs

KFC Creamy Parmesan Caesar: 4g net carbs

Heinz Buttermilk Ranch: 1g net carbs

McDonald's

All of the McDonald's low-carb options take out the bun or bread (biscuit, muffins) and have no ketchup included. The buns alone on the burgers account for more than ¾ of the carb count listed on the nutrition facts!

Breakfast: There really aren't a whole lot of low-carb options for breakfast since most of their famous breakfast options include muffins, biscuits, and/or syrup.

Modified Egg McMuffin: take out the muffin, keep the egg, American cheese, and ham or sausage and it goes from about 30g net carbs to 2.

Basically, any other item on the breakfast menu would follow the same rules: take out bread and sauces and stay away from the hash browns!

Burgers/Sandwiches: Again, follow these simple rules: no bread or condiments (except for mustard), get them wrapped in lettuce instead. All the meats (as long as they're dry) have 0g net carbs and almost all of the toppings have 0-1g net carbs. Absolutely no fries!

Some good low carb options are:

Big Mac (dry no buns): 6g net carbs

Quarter Pounder w/ Cheese (dry, no buns): 7g net carbs

Bacon Clubhouse Burger (dry, no buns): 8g net carbs

Grilled Chicken (dry, no bun): 2g net carbs

Filet-o-Fish (dry, no bun): splurge w/ cheese a side of tartar sauce comes to about 10g net carbs

Salads

Side Salads (no dressing): 2g net carbs

Caesar w/ Grilled Chicken (no croutons): 9g net carbs

Bacon Ranch w/ Grilled Chicken: 6g net carbs

Dressing Packets

Creamy Caesar: 4g net carbs

Low Fat Balsamic Vinaigrette: 6g net carbs

Ranch: 2-4g net carbs

Taco Bell

Taco Bell doesn't have a specifically low-carb menu either, but here are some options for making some of the regular menu items keto friendly. If you're stressing and feel like you just can't find anything, simply removing beans, potatoes, and rice from dishes will dramatically reduce carbs. All hot sauces are 0g net carbs.

Breakfast

Mini Skillet Bowl- with eggs, pico de gallo and nacho cheese (hold the potatoes): 3g net carbs

Power Menu Bowls

Steak Power Bowl (hold beans and rice): 1g net carbs

Ground Beef Power Bowl (hold beans and rice): 7g net carbs

Chicken Power Bowl (hold beans and rice): 5g net carbs

Add-Ons (all 0-2g net carbs)

Steak: 1g net carb

Fire Grilled Chicken: 0g net carbs

Shredded Chicken: 1g net carbs

Seasoned Ground Beef: 1g net carbs

Guacamole: 1,5g net carbs

Bacon: 0g net carbs

Shredded Cheddar: 0g net carbs

Sausage Crumbles: 0g net carbs

Shredded 3 Cheese Blend: 0g net carbs

Sour Cream: 2g net carbs

Extra Cheese Sauce: 2g net carbs

Jalapenos: 0.5g net carbs

Chipotle

Chipotle is a little more health/low-carb friendly than some of the other fast food choices without technically having the options on the menu. They make an effort to keep their ingredients fresh and just about anything on their menu can be made as a salad, which is going to be the best keto option.

For the salad bowls, you can get any of the meats (steak, chicken, pork, barbacoa), cheese, sour cream (make sure it's full fat), red salsa, and guacamole. Steer clear of corn and the green salsas and mix and match all you want!

Sizzler

The buffet side of Sizzler is potentially very dangerous for a keto diet even though it's just a salad bar. There are some very good choices on their menus for keto entrees, but you will have to be careful with the salad bar.

Salads

Asian Chopped Salad (1/2 cup): 3g net carbs

Cucumber Tomato Salad (1/2 cup): 4g net carbs

Greek Salad (1/2 cup): 1g net carbs

Main Dishes

Grilled Salmon w/ Vegetable Medley (6oz, no tartar sauce): 10g net carbs

Italian Herbed Chicken w/ Steamed Broccoli: 9g net carbs

Hibachi Chicken w/ Steamed Broccoli: 12g net carbs (Note: get without sauces and pineapple to bring carb count down)

Shrimp Skewers w/ Cilantro Rice & Steamed Broccoli: 33g net carbs (Note: this is a pretty high carb count! Asking for no rice will bring it down considerably, also request no garlic margarine.)

South Atlantic Red Shrimp Skewers w/ Steamed Broccoli: 42g net carbs (Note: this dish also comes with cilantro rice; no rice will bring carb count down.)

Shrimp Skewers w/ Cilantro Rice and Vegetable Medley: 34g net carbs (Note: another higher carb dish; get it without rice and garlic margarine.)

Tri Tip Steak w/ Vegetable Medley (6oz steak): 8g net carbs

Sides

Tri-Color Quinoa Kale Salad: 13g net carbs (Note: Quinoa is high in protein; if you choose this, make sure you are monitoring protein intake for the rest of the day.)

Steamed Broccoli: 7g net carbs

Vegetable Medley: 8g net carbs

Subway

Obviously, sandwiches are out! But thankfully Subway will make most of their sandwiches as salads that can be tweaked to make them more filling and with the right amount of fat. You can add veggies, usually with no extra charge, or ask for double the meat. You will most likely have to pay for that, but it will make the salads more filling.

Chopped Tuna Salad w/ oil & vinegar (get with extra bacon!): 2g net carbs

Spicy Italian Chopped Salad: 5g net carbs

Cold Cut Combo Salad: 5g net carbs

Subway Club Salad w/ oil & vinegar (double the meat): 5g net carbs

Italian BMT Salad (double the meat): 5g net carbs

Roasted Chicken Patty Salad w/ oil & vinegar: 3g net carbs

Red Robin

If it's burgers you want, the easiest way to keep it Keto is to skip the bun and wrap them in lettuce. Forgo most sauces and condiments or ask for them on the side. You can add bacon for 0g net carbs or cheese for only 1g net carbs.

Wedgie Burger: Red Robin actually does have a specifically low-carb meal on their menu and it's called the Wedgie Burger. It comes on a lettuce wedge and includes bacon, guacamole, tomato, and onion. If you don't want the beef patty you can substitute it with a chicken or turkey burger.

Bottomless Salad: Red Robin is famous for their bottomless fries and thankfully you can swap the fries out for bottomless salad.

Wedge Salad: Their wedge salad is constructed the same way as the Wedgie Burger, just without the burger meat. It is a wedge of iceberg lettuce topped with blue cheese, tomatoes, bacon bits, and onion straws. Skip the onions to make it keto appropriate.

Golden Corral

Buffet style restaurants could make it more difficult to be disciplined. One of the upsides, however, is the fact that you get to fill your own plate. You don't have to feel like you're inconveniencing the servers and chefs. Here are some low-carb meal ideas from Golden Corral. Keep in mind: according to their nutrition facts, quite a few of their dishes contain wheat and soy.

Breakfast: There are not an abundance of keto friendly breakfasts at Golden Corral, but they do have some low-carb breakfast staples you can mix and match to create a meal.

Bacon: 3 pieces= 0g net carbs

Chorizo & Eggs: ½ cup serving= 2g net carbs

Made-To-Order Eggs: 1 egg= 1g net carbs

Sausage: 1 link= 1g net carbs

Meat Dishes: Golden Corral has countless meats prepared in a variety of different ways. Not all of them are keto friendly due to how they're prepared. Here are a few that are good for low-carb diets that don't contain wheat and/or soy.

Garlic Herb Butter Sirloin: 3oz= 1g net carbs

Garlic Parmesan Sirloin: 3oz= 1g net carbs

Lemon Rosemary Sirloin: 3oz= 1g net carbs

Rib Eye: 3oz= 0g net carbs

Boneless Chicken Wings w/ Frank's Hot Sauce: 3 pieces= 0g net carbs

Rotisserie Chicken: 1 piece= 1g net carbs

Baby Back Pork Ribs: 1 rib= 3g net carbs

BBQ Pork: 3oz= 4g net carbs

Grilled Ham Steaks: 2 pieces= 5g net carbs

Seafood: All the seafood dishes contain soy and wheat; it would best to steer clear of those.

Sides: All of the sides either contain wheat and soy or are too high in carbs to be keto friendly.

Vegetables

Steamed Broccoli: ½ cup= 3g net carbs

Steamed Cauliflower: ½ cup= 1g net carbs

Sautéed Spinach: ½ cup= 1g net carbs

Vegetable Trio: ½ cup= 4g net carbs

Dairy Queen

Obviously, the ice cream is off limits. But some of the regular menu favorites can be modified into low-carb options.

Turkey BLT (without ciabatta roll): Sliced turkey, melted Swiss cheese, bacon, lettuce, tomato, and mayo. Hold off on the mayo to bring carbs down even more: 3g net carbs

Original Cheeseburger (without the bun): Beef patty, lettuce, American cheese, pickles, onions and mustard. Only add mayo if you need the extra fat: 3g net carbs

Grilled Chicken BLT Salad: Bacon, chicken, cheese, lettuce, and ranch dressing: without dressing= 7g net carbs, with dressing= 10g net carbs

FlameThrower GrillBurger (without the bun, spicy!): Either one half pound patty or (depending on location) two quarter pound patties, creamy jalapeno sauce, jalapeno bacon, lettuce, sliced jalapeños, tomato, and pepper jack: 4g net carbs

Chicken Bacon Ranch (without ciabatta roll): Chicken breasts, tomato, lettuce, melted Swiss, ranch, and bacon: 5g net carbs

Starbucks (Food Only)

Starbucks has developed a good balance of keeping classic food selections and bringing in new ones. They seem to have focused more on low or reduced fat options, but there are a couple of things that can be eaten on a keto diet. Note: "reduced fat" items are not keto options.

Breakfast

Sous Vide Egg Bites: Rich and yummy, these are technically keto friendly but they are on the high end of the carb spectrum, so keep track of carb intake the rest of the day: 9g net carbs per order

Snacks

Snack Boxes: the protein box does include a hard-boiled egg and some cheese, but the rest of the contents aren't keto friendly.

Kind Bars: These are keto friendly, but they are also high in carbs (8g) and they're not even a full meal.

Wingstop

Chicken is definitely a must have for keto diets, but not all forms are healthy. Here are some wing options at Wingstop that are keto friendly. Note: the info listed below is based on an order of 10 wings.

Plain Wings: 0g net carbs

Atomic: 5g net carbs

Mild: 0g net carbs

Garlic Parmesan: 0g net carbs

Cajon: 0g net carbs

Original (hot!): 0g net carbs

Louisiana Rub: 0g net carbs

Lemon Pepper: 0g net carbs

Pair the wings with ranch or blue cheese and celery sticks!

Cheesecake Factory

This chain is absolutely a family favorite! Most of the menu, unfortunately, is not keto friendly but there are a few meals that fit the carb requirements.

Starters: Almost all of the starters are upwards of 30g net carbs and more. The carpaccio is the one option that might have a low enough carb count to work: 11g net carbs (serves 2).

Salads (small options)

Boston House Salad: 11g net carbs

BLT Salad: 15g net carbs

Caesar Salad (with or without chicken): Less than 20g net carbs

Cobb Salad (lunch side): Less than 20g net carbs

Entrees (will have to be modified)

Sandwiches and burgers: order them dry, without the bun/bread

Steak, Seafood, Sides

One option outside of modifying meals on your own is taking advantage of Cheesecake Factory's make-your-own meals. Choose as low carb meats and sides as you can.

Steak Diane: 10g net carbs

Petite Rib Eye: 24g net carbs

Petite Fillet: 23g net carbs

Grilled Salmon: 3g net carbs

Grilled Tuna: 3g net carbs

Grilled Mahi Mahi: 3g net carbs

Herb-Crusted Salmon: 8g net carbs

Green Beans (side): 6g net carbs

Sautéed Spinach (side): 6g net carbs

Asparagus (side): 7g net carbs

Broccoli (side): 9g net carbs

Olive Garden

Italian restaurants can be daunting for any dieter, and there really aren't many low-carb options available. But they do have a few and they even have their own spot on the menu.

Salads & Sides:

Fresh Spinach Salad: 3g net carbs

Oven Roasted Asparagus: 1g net carbs

Bottomless Salad: essentially everything in this salad is keto friendly; even the dressing, up to a certain amount. If you're going that route, ask for a cup of dressing on the side.

Entrees

Herb Grilled Salmon & Broccoli: 1g net carbs

Jason Michaels & Thomas Hawthorn

Steak Toscano & Grilled Vegetables: 32g net carbs

Mixed Grill Steak & Chicken Skewers with Grilled Vegetables: 20g net carbs

Alfredo sauce is actually fairly low carb so you can order a side of that for your veggies if you need to make the meal more interesting.

Five Guys Burgers

Five Guys has actually gone out of their way to make their menu low-carb optional, which definitely makes them stand out from the average fast food place. You can literally get any burger on the menu either bunless or in a tin salad-style. You can get the works, all of which are acceptable, except for the ketchup and maybe the mayo unless you need the fat. Here are just a few of the options Five Guys offers. The milkshakes are off limits!

Bunless Hot Dog in a Tin: with relish, onions, and mustard: 7g net carbs

Cheeseburger in a Lettuce Wrap: 1g net carbs

Bunless Bacon Double Cheeseburger in a Tin: try it with jalapeños, bacon, and cheese: 2g net carbs

In-N-Out

In-N-Out has also made an effort to offer low carb choices. They have an entire hidden menu; not all of them are low-carb but a few of them are. Ask for any of the burger protein style to skip the bun and get them wrapped in lettuce.

Double Double Protein Style: two patties, two slices of cheese, special sauce, and all the toppings: 8g net carbs

Cheeseburger Protein Style: single patty, single cheese, special sauce, and all the toppings: 8g net carbs

Hamburger Animal and Protein Style (secret menu): all the burgers can be ordered animal style; it just means the burger is fried in mustard and then they add grilled onions, more pickles, and extra special sauce: 11g net carbs

4x4 Cheeseburger Protein Style (secret menu): four patties, four slices of cheese, two slices of tomato, special sauce: 8g net carbs

3x3 Cheeseburger Protein Style (secret menu): exactly the same as the "quad" but with one less patty, etc.: 8g net carbs

Panera

Although Panera specializes in bread, pastries, and sandwiches, much of their menu can simply be ordered without the bread. They also have a selection of soups and salads that can be keto friendly.

Breakfast: Basically any of their breakfast sandwiches can be ordered without the bread and still function as a satisfying meal.

Ham, Egg, & Cheese Sandwich (without bread): 3g net carbs

Turkey Sausage, Egg White, & Spinach Sandwich (without bread): 2g net carbs

Sausage, Egg, & Cheese Sandwich (without the bread): 3g net carbs

Steak, Egg, & Cheese Bagel Sandwich (without the bagel): 3g net carbs

Lunch & Dinner

Steak & Baby Arugula Sandwich (on lettuce): 10g net carbs

Caesar Chicken Salad (without croutons): 6g net carbs

Green Goddess Cobb Salad (add chicken): 10g net carbs

Italian Sandwich (without bread): ham, sopressa, salami, arugula, provolone, giardiniera, and basil mayo (get the mayo on the side): 4g net carbs

Steak & White Cheddar (without bread): on a bed of lettuce: 7g net carbs

Roasted Turkey & Avocado BLT (without bread): 2g net carbs

Whataburger

Whataburger is yet another burger chain with a menu that can be easily modified into low-carb meals. Here are just a few examples of how to make these burgers keto friendly.

Breakfast

Sausage, Egg, & Cheese Sandwich (without bun): 0g net carbs

Scrambled Eggs & Bacon (3 slices of bacon): 3g net carbs

Sausage, Egg, & Cheese Taquito (no tortilla): 3g net carbs

Lunch & Dinner

Double Meat Whataburger add Double Cheese, Bacon, & Jalapeno (without the bun): 5g net carbs (add a side of ranch for about 1 additional g of net carbs)

Grilled Chicken Melt w/ Lettuce (without the bun): 3g net carbs

Whataburger Patty Melt (without the bun): 2g net carbs

Garden Salad w/ Whatachik'n: 17g net carbs- to reduce carb count, get without the fried chicken and take off tomatoes and carrots. Ranch dressing adds about 1g additional net carb.

Cracker Barrel

Jason Michaels *&* Thomas Hawthorn

This restaurant will forever be a family favorite with its great vibe and scrumptious down home meals. Cracker Barrel has also added some great low carb option to their menu.

Breakfast

Country Grilled Sampler: bacon, sausage, sliced tomatoes, and country ham: 4g net carbs (no toast, drop the tomatoes to lower carb count if needed)

Double Meat Breakfast: three eggs, sausage, bacon, and sliced tomatoes (no toast, drop tomatoes if needed).

Eggs 'n Meat: three eggs, sausage or bacon, and sliced tomatoes: 2 net carbs (no toast, drop tomatoes if needed).

Lunch or Dinner

Grilled Steak Salad: 7g net carbs (not including dressing)

Lemon Pepper Grilled Trout: 0g net carbs (not counting sides)

Half Pound Bacon Cheeseburger (no bun): 3g net carbs (not counting sides)

Grilled Roast Beef: 4g net carbs (not counting sides)

Sides

Blue Cheese Dressing: 2g net carbs

Buttermilk Ranch: 1g net carbs

Spicy Pork Rinds: 1g net carbs

Green Beans: 2g net carbs

Texas Roadhouse

Texas Roadhouse is a very popular steakhouse. Thankfully, with these types of restaurants, the options to order low-carb are fairly plentiful. Between the numerous steak dishes and their choice of salads, staying in ketosis should be a cinch at this restaurant.

Starters

Boneless Buffalo Wings (Hot Sauce): 8g net carbs

Boneless Buffalo Wings (Mild Sauce): 8g net carbs

Texas Red Chili (cup): 7g net carbs

Note: the bowl is considerably higher in carbs; if you are planning on eating an entrée as well, the cup would be the best option.

Salads

California Chicken Salad (meal size): 12g net carbs

Chicken Caesar (meal size, with dressing): 16g net carbs

Grilled Chicken (meal size): 13g net carbs

Grilled Salmon (meal size): 11g net carbs

Caesar (side): 9g net carbs

House Salad (side): 7g net carbs

Dressings

Blue Cheese (2oz): 4g net carbs

Ranch (2oz): 4g net carbs

Caesar (2oz): 4g net carbs

Steak Options (10g and under)

Dallas Filet (6oz): 4g net carbs

Dallas Filet (8oz): 6g net carbs

Ft. Worth Ribeye (10oz, 12oz, 16oz): 0g net carbs

New York/Kansas City Strip (8oz, 12oz): 1g net carbs

Prime Rib (10oz, 12oz): 5g net carbs

Chicken Options (10g and under)

Oven Roasted Half Chicken: 7g net carbs

Portobello Mushroom Chicken: 7g net carbs

Country Dinners (Pork)

Grilled Pork Chops (single): 3g net carbs

Grilled Pork Chops (double): 6g net carbs

Fish

Grilled Salmon (5oz, 8oz): 1g net carbs

Sides

Jason Michaels & Thomas Hawthorn

Fresh Vegetables: 7g net carbs

Sautéed Mushrooms: 4g net carbs

Green Beans: 11g net carbs

Red Lobster

Seafood is fairly versatile as well. Many of the dishes are paired with butter sauces, which should be keto friendly. And they have a handy low-carb section on their menu to make ordering easy. And, as heart breaking as it is, you'll have to forgo the classic, addicting cheddar biscuits.

Starters

Buffalo Chicken Wings: 4g net carbs

Shellfish Dishes

Shrimp Your Way (Scampi): 3g net carbs

Wild-Caught Snow Crab Legs: 0g net carbs

Live Maine Lobster (1.25lb, steamed): 0g net carbs

Feasts & Combos

CYO-Garlic Shrimp Scampi: 3g net carbs

CYO- Fresh Wood-Grilled Tilapia: 1g net carbs

CYO- Wood Grilled Sea Scallops: 4g net carbs

CYO- 7oz Wood-Grilled Sirloin: 1g net carbs

Other Fish Dishes

Salmon New Orleans (half or full): 8g net carbs

Wild-Caught Flounder (oven broiled): 1g net carbs

Sides & Salads (under 10g net carbs)

Garden Salad: 9g net carbs

Fresh Asparagus: 2g net carbs

Grilled Shrimp (add to salad): 0g net carbs

Fresh Broccoli: 5g net carbs

Classic Lunch Dishes

Farm-Raised Blackened Catfish: 2g net carbs

Chapter 2: Keto Options at Generic Non-Chain/Mom & Pop Restaurants

Some of the best meals we've ever had have come from quaint little "mom & and pop" restaurants, many of them offering a variety of ethnic foods. They may not be big chain franchises but they make up for it with nostalgia and good food. One of the negatives of these dining establishments is that nutrition details will probably be much harder to come by. There are still plenty of options for making meals low-carb, they just won't be as easily accessible on the menu. If you find you are having trouble putting together a low-carb meal, it's never wrong to politely ask an establishment how some of their menu items are prepared. Here are some tips on how to make some of these ethnic and generic restaurant foods more keto friendly.

Italian

Whenever we think "Italian food", we immediately imagine pasta, bread, pizza, cheese, more bread...so, essentially, carb heaven! Italian food is easily a favorite for many people, and initially, it may seem that low-carb choices will be impossible to find. Thankfully, that is not the case.

Pasta and pizza are very much staples in Italian food restaurants here in America and a big part of these dishes are the toppings, which usually consist of good meats and healthy veggies. Try ordering a pasta or pizza meal but ask for the toppings to go over lettuce. If you can, make sure the vegetables are cooked in olive oil, or even butter, if it's full fat. Grass fed is preferable but not always attainable. Opt for straight olive oil and vinegar for the dressing, unless you've confirmed that their ranch or Caesar does not have excess amounts of sugar, especially if it's house-made.

Grilled chicken, beef, or fish will also most likely be on the menu, you'll just have to forgo carb-loaded sides and sauces. Pesto is an option to spread over chicken but use sparingly because of the pine nuts.

Antipasto ("before meal") platters are often available for appetizers. These plates usually consist of meats, vegetables, and sometimes seafood, all of which are excellent low-carb options.

Soups can be a good keto meal as well, as long as they are made with thinner broths rather than thicker "chowder" bases. Chowders often need starch and/or flour to make them thicken which will knock you out of ketosis very quickly. Steer clear of soups with pasta, beans, or gnocchi in them as well.

Mexican

Mexican cuisine is delicious and exciting, but much of it includes beans and rice in a variety of forms witch is not conducive to staying in ketosis. Requesting meals without the rice and beans will immediately lower the carb count.

You can get just about any meal that comes in a tortilla either on the side or over a bed of shredded lettuce. Cheese, full fat sour cream, red salsas, and avocado are all keto approved. Watch out for the additives in guacamole. If you would rather have that over plain avocado slices, be sure to ask what the ingredients are.

Any meat that is grilled is fine and you can even request it over fajita-grilled vegetables rather than inside of a tortilla. Sides such as ceviche and pico de gallo are also options for spicing up your modified meal.

Japanese/Sushi

A lot of Japanese and sushi dishes already cater to low-carb diets with little to no modification. Granted, sushi does come with rice so sashimi is a better choice. Avoid edamame as well; ½ a cup of those little guys easily reaches 9-10g net carbs!

Miso soup is a good low-carb choice. It is a good keto friendly starter and will help fill you up if you find you have limited keto options. Some Japanese restaurants have a dish called Konjac Ramen, which is one of the few noodle-type dishes that will be low-carb enough for your diet. The noodles are made out of the root of the elephant yam and the single serving size only comes to about 2-3g net carbs. Granted, there are other toppings on ramen bowls, so you will have to be conscientious about the other ingredients to keep it low carb.

As with the other restaurants, grilled meats are always a good choice provided they are not covered in any kind of sauce. Non-seafood options at sushi restaurants often consist of either beef or chicken teriyaki bowls. You could modify these by getting the sauce on the side and forgoing the rice.

Indian

Indian cuisine might be a bit more difficult to get low-carb options for. While the spices are very good, many of the dishes come with sauces and unless you're making it yourself, it could be difficult to find any without sugars or flours used to thicken them. Try to order meat dishes, with little to no sauce if possible, and always skip the naan and rice.

Tandoori chicken can be a good choice; just keep in mind tandoori marinade usually contains yogurt, a lot of which is not very low-carb. Also, any kind of kabobs with meat and veggies are good as long as the meat is dry.

BBQ

Once of the biggest carb hang-ups, you'll come across at a BBQ joint is the sauces. Asking for your baby back ribs with no sauce does seem like it defeats the purpose. But BBQ restaurants are all about the smoking and the seasoning as well. A well-seasoned dry rubbed steak or rack of ribs will be just as enjoyable without the sauce. If asking for no sauce seems like a big deal you can always request it on the side. Sadly, just about every version of a BBQ sauce will be off limits due to the high amount of sugar, even in house-made sauces.

Also try to avoid pre-sauced dishes like pulled pork, barbacoa, or other shredded meats that are prepared in the sauce. Some southern BBQ places might use a sauce made with vinegar and mustard, which will be keto friendly.

If you're ordering wings, ask if there is a dry rub version (like they offer at Buffalo Wild Wings) or simply get them dry with buffalo sauce on the side. Pair them with ranch or blue cheese and celery sticks (try to avoid starchy carrots).

The same salad and side rules apply here as any other restaurant; steer clear of sweet, fruity dressings, hold the croutons, no bread or fried sides!

Sports Bars

Sports bars will probably have similar choices to chains like Applebee's, Chili's, and Buffalo Wild Wings, with the exception of limited nutrition facts and a few low carb choices on the menus. Still, the same concepts work for these non-chain restaurants.

If you're hanging with friends watching the big game, it's easy to just start munching on whatever lands on the table while you watch. Order all of your own appetizers and entrees rather than sharing orders with others who don't have the same diet requirements.

Steak is always a win, which will mostly likely be one of the options on the menu at a sports bar. The same goes for chicken, as long as it's not breaded. Grilled fish, pork chops, and bunless burgers are wise choices as well. Again, be mindful of sides and swap out dippable veggies like cucumbers and celery for the fries or potatoes.

Chapter 3: Keto Options at Convenience Stores & Gas Stations

Let's face it...we all need vacations in our lives! Figuring out what to eat once you're at your destination is one problem. What to eat along the way is another. Any long road trip or even time spent in an airport is going to require a pit stop of some kind. These stops are usually at stores with nothing but chips and candy...or so it seems. Even if there is no road trip involved, a quick trip to a 7/11 store to satisfy the "munchies" could be dangerous ground. Here are some quick, easy, and Keto friendly finds.

Cheese

Yes, cheese is our friend; and a very low-carb, fulfilling snack for on the go. You can get mozzarella string cheese or even jack or cheddar cheeses that come in a similar form. Make sure they are full fat and limit yourself to one or two to keep carbs down.

Raw Vegetables

Many convenience and gas station stores have small refrigerated sections where you can find great keto options, like raw veggies. Try to pick celery or broccoli over carrots and get a ranch dressing packet to go with it. Steer clear of peanut butter and hummus.

Hard Boiled Eggs

Perhaps not every convenience store will have these, but bigger ones like Walgreens or 7/11 might. These are the perfect keto snack and if the egg isn't enough you could even pair it with the veggies.

Cold Cuts

You might also find some cold cuts in the refrigerated section. Take care to read the ingredients, however. Some may be packed with sugary or really high sodium extras. These would also go well with the veggies and boiled eggs.

Jerky

Jerky is definitely an American staple! It is a great source of protein, and you can find it literally anywhere. Poultry jerkies will have less fat than beef, so go with the beef if you need to up your fat intake. Look at the ingredients before you buy it to make sure there aren't any added sugars and get original rather than flavored, like teriyaki.

Pork Rinds

These suckers have been around forever and have taken the keto world by storm! These are an excellent choice if you just need something to munch and you can even dip them in ranch or blue cheese if you need to.

Kale Chips

Kale chips are a fairly new addition to the convenience store roster and not every establishment will have them. If you find a store along the way that sells them, you might want to stock up for the rest of your trip. They are also an excellent substitute for chips or pretzels and can effectively satisfy the need to munch.

Hot Dogs

Any convenience store and most gas station stores will have a hot food section, with items like burritos, burgers, and hot dogs. The burgers will probably come already in the bun but the dogs are usually kept hot on their own. Grab one or two, skip the bun, add some mustard or ranch, and you have a Keto snack to go along with your veggies or kale chips.

Chapter 4: Keto Options: Low Carb Alcoholic & Coffee Beverages

For some, giving up alcohol or coffee may not be so bad. For others, it would be the end of the world! Have no fear; there are easily accessible low-carb options both at restaurants and coffee shops.

Keto Friendly Alcoholic Options

Wine & Beer: If you have to choose between one or the other, wines and champagnes have much fewer carbs than beer. Plus, beer is wheat based which will take your body out of ketosis very quickly.

For a keto diet, even if you're trying to stay below 20g net carbs a day, a glass of wine somewhat regularly would be alright. Try to choose dry wines as they will contain 0.5g sugar and under per glass. Definitely avoid ports and other sweet dessert wines. If there is not a suitable wine choice at the restaurant you might have to search for an alternative.

Beer is basically off limits period if you're trying to stay in ketosis unless you order very light American beers. But if you absolutely need a beer and the restaurant has very low carb choices, then you can safely have one on occasion if needed.

Spirits: Straight spirits are all 0g net carbs. It's the stuff that gets added to them you have to watch out for. For example, a vodka and soda water (aka "skinny bitch") is 0g net carbs while a Bloody Mary with vodka is 7g. When ordering mixed cocktails, avoid the ones with added sugars from syrups, sodas, and liqueurs. Dry martinis are also low-carb

Wine Coolers & Alcopops: all of these are off limits for keto diets. They are loaded with sugar; you're basically drinking a soda with some alcohol in it.

Keto Friendly Coffee Beverages

We all have that one friend who you would never want to meet in a dark alley on a caffeine rage. Or maybe you are that friend! Coffee is a staple for many to live through the day and it is very easy to find keto approved coffee beverages.

Starbucks Keto Drinks

Starbucks is probably the most well-known and widespread coffee chain in the world. They may not have too much going on for low-carb meals, but their keto coffee choices are quite vast and delicious.

Black Coffee: This one is kind of a no-brainer; if you want your coffee as low-carb as possibly, drink it black! Americanos are very low-carb as well.

Low-Carb Mocha: Replace the milk in the regular mocha with half water and half heavy cream. Ask for the skinny mocha sauce instead of regular.

Low-Carb Flat White: Replace steamed milk with half water, half heavy cream and you will maintain the creamy texture while cutting out much of the carbs.

Low-Carb Misto: Replace the milk with half and half water/heavy cream. Order it "short" and it will have only 5g net carbs (without modifications).

Low-Carb Vanilla Latte: Replace the milk with water/heavy cream and ask for sugar-free vanilla syrup.

Obviously, Starbucks is a coffee shop and can afford to be versatile. Ordering keto friendly coffee in fast food or sit down restaurants may be more difficult. When in doubt, always order it in black. If you have the option, get heavy cream instead of creamer. Or, you can bring your own MCT oil if it's the fatty taste you're craving. Use the Starbucks guidelines for ordering espresso drinks at other establishments and beware of the syrups! If you have to have the syrup make sure it's always sugar free and you have substituted the milk for heavy cream.

Side note: all teas without honey or sugar are low carb, so knock yourself out!

Chapter 5: Keto Imposters &"Contraband"

If you feel like you have been sticking to the diet but are failing to see results, you may have been consuming "hidden" carbs and might have dropped out of ketosis.

Keto Imposters

There are the obvious slip-ups in sodas and candy. But even some reportedly healthy foods are not keto friendly at all. Cereals are some of the biggest imposters: 1 cup of cheerios has 17g net carbs, 1 cup of GoLean Crunch has 22g net carbs, Special K has 22g, and shredded wheat has a whopping 39g net carbs in a 1 cup serving!

Health or protein bars can also hide carbs. The chocolate chip Clif Bar alone has 41g net carbs! That's almost double the number of carbs in 1 serving that you should be eating in all your meals for one day on the keto diet.

Many Keto diet shopping lists include some fruits and nuts. In reality, most if not all should be avoided while trying to stay in ketosis. They are just too high in carbs to compensate for the fats and proteins they might be able to offer. The same goes for beans and legumes. If you have to have fruit in your life, choose low sugar berries such as blackberries, raspberries, or blueberries (try to keep serving sizes at ½ a cup or under).

Vegetables are definitely on the list, but not every vegetable is created equal. Take care limit and/or avoid starchy veggies such as sweet potatoes, regular potatoes, corn, carrots, peas, and even cherry tomatoes.

Sugars are an obvious no-no, but they often creep up even in foods we thought were healthy and keto friendly. Even "healthy" sugars can kick your body out of ketosis. Pay close attention to nutrition facts and try to avoid even natural sugars found in honey, syrups, raw sugar, agave nectar, and cane sugar.

Dairy is listed on Keto diets but still should be consumed in moderation and always full fat. Some dairy products that are not actually keto friendly are: low fat or 2% milks, low fat cottage cheese, pre-packaged shredded cheeses (which often include potato starch), low fat or substitute butters, and yogurts (both low and full fat as it is really hard to find low carb/sugar yogurts).

Keto Contraband

The keto diet could be described as fairly easy in, very easy out. In other words, it's not too difficult to go into ketosis (usually depending on what method you use) but it also doesn't take much to go out of it again. Part of making a lifestyle change includes kicking bad habits and cutting out bad foods...sometimes forever. The Keto diet may be temporarily based on your goals and health needs, and some foods may be "borderline" contraband. But if you're trying to remain in ketosis for any extended amount of time without having to start the process over, here are some foods to avoid at all costs in order to stay on track.

Some of the obvious ones that will kick your body out of ketosis are potatoes, all bread and grains (including pasta, even whole wheat), rice, beer, sodas, and juice, low fat dairy products, and yogurt.

Any coffee additives that are artificial (like creamers and sugars) should be avoided as well as cheese spread and some salad dressings. Many commercially made dressings, even potentially keto approved ones, have tons of added sugars. Steer clear of any fruit based dressings (such as berry vinaigrettes) and especially any labeled "low" or "reduced" fat; it's the fat you want, just not the carbs.

Most types of gravy and sauces are flour based to make them thicker and have added sugars for flavors. Finding any that are specifically low-carb at restaurants will be practically impossible, so it's best to always skip sauces and gravy when eating out if you want to stay in ketosis.

As we discussed earlier, there are a very few choices of fruit that are Keto friendly. Most of them should be avoided at all costs, due to their very high carb counts. These include Apples, kiwis, cherries, grapes, bananas, mangos, and citrus fruits.

Desserts that are sugary and/or bread and wheat based are also naturally off limits, such as candy and chocolate (unless it's at least 70% dark cacao), donuts, cakes, muffins, cupcakes, cake pops, and ice cream (unless it's specifically Keto friendly).

Chapter 6: Helpful Tips & Guidelines

One of the many perks of the Keto diet is, it has very few rules. There are so many foods you can eat (that taste great) and it fits perfectly into just about any exercise or training routine. That being said, there are some general easy-to-follow rules that will help you keep your body in ketosis when ordering food on the go.

Meats, Cheese, & Veggies

When in doubt, keep it simple! You won't always be able to quickly find pertinent nutrition facts at a restaurant, so sticking to these basics will keep you safe. Get your meat without sauces, especially if you can't find out if they have added sugars or not. Natural cheeses are preferable over American cheese, but either is fine. Ask for your veggies to be sautéed in butter if you don't like them steamed. Granted, this request may not fly at every dining spot, but many restaurants are happy to accommodate.

No Buns!

Bread is a sure way to carb load too much and knock your body out of ketosis. Even whole grains have a lot of sugar binding lectins in them. If you absolutely have to have bread and the restaurant can provide it, go with sprouted grains. But, the easiest option here is really to request the sandwich or burger wrapped in lettuce or served salad-style. Add-ons such as bacon or avocado will help satisfy you and ease the loss of the bread. Many sauces and condiments are keto appropriate; just make sure to keep an eye on the sugar content!

If ordering a salad (whether it started that way or you're creating your own) make sure to take into account all of the ingredients! Just because it's a salad, it doesn't mean you're always in the clear. Many salads come with croutons, nuts, or fruit, and high carb dressings. Even some leafy greens are higher in carbs. Go for salads that have meat in them to ensure you are getting enough fats and protein and when in doubt, get the dressing on the side. Greek restaurants are a good place to find delicious low-carb gyro-style salads. Skip all croutons and other carby/sugary ingredients and toppings.

Skip the Breading

The same concept for skipping buns goes for breading on fried foods as well if the breading is wheat based. If you really want what's underneath the breading, it's usually pretty easy to peel it off. You can then pair it with a fatty sauce like ranch or buffalo sauce. Or, you might even be able to order the dish without the breading (chicken wings, for example). There are keto-friendly breading options, such as crushed pork rinds, low-carb breadcrumbs, and parmesan and seasonings, but these types of breading will probably be difficult to impossible to find on a menu or even as a special request. It's always nice when the restaurant is accommodating, but we have to remember to not take it too far.

Watch Out for Condiments

Like we mentioned above, a vast majority of condiments and sauces are loaded with sugars and possibly even an overabundance of sodium (too much of a good thing and all that). Still, it is possible to use condiments and sauces to add flavor without getting into trouble. Any sweet-tasting sauces or dressings (like Teriyaki sauces or BBQ sauce) definitely have too much sugar for keto diets. Stick to fattier dressing and sauces like ranch (dressing or dip), buffalo sauce, sour cream (full fat), blue cheese, and Caesar. Keep in mind, some Caesar dressings are more sugary than others, so keep an eye on nutrition facts if possible. Plain yellow mustard is also a keto safe condiment and you could even ask for sides of butter if needed to get your daily fat intake up.

Making Special Requests

For some, the thought of being "that person" makes us squirm. But, at the end of the day, you have a responsibility to take care of yourself and as long as you keep requests respectful and attainable, you should have relatively little pushback. You should prepare yourself for some discomfort, but don't let that interfere with your health goals.

It's pretty standard these days to request burgers at fast food places without the bun; some joints even have these options on the main menu. Nutrition facts are also now readily available at any restaurant making it easier to quickly customize meal choices. You're more likely to get confused or irritated responses from employees for special requests made at fast food restaurants, so try to keep these as simple as possible. Asking for a burger "protein style" or lettuce wrapped is common enough. Don't give a long list of what you want or don't want; ask for cheese if you want cheese, specify toppings, then just get it dry. You can most likely get ranch and/or mustard easily enough on the side when you pick up your order. Be prepared for screw-ups on fast food special orders...it's just how it goes...and be grateful when they do get it right!

At sit down restaurants, you will be able to request more sophisticated alterations. It's actually pretty common to ask for no added salt to your meal and most sit down and family restaurants (chains especially) now have lite or low-carb sections in their menus. Those options make it much easier to get Keto appropriate meals without having to make special requests. Still, it is important to pay attention to additives listed in nutrition facts and sides that come with a meal. A grilled chicken dish is always a good low-carb choice. If it comes with steamed or even sautéed veggies, as long as butter or olive oil is used. However, these dishes are often served with rice, potatoes, and/or bread as well, which are definitely not Keto friendly. The a la carte options on menus could solve this problem well; you could always add a house salad to make the meal more complete. Keep in mind, however, this could also be a more expensive option. Chances are you could get the meal and opt out of those sides and even ask for double veggies to keep it filling.

Conclusion

Thanks for making it through to the end of Keto Diet on the Go, let's hope it was informative and able to provide you with all of the tools you need to achieve your goals whatever they may be.

The next step is to not be afraid to ask for low-carb options and to try new things. There are times when we fall into ruts when we start new routines because it's comfortable and easier to handle. Starting and sustaining a keto diet may not take as much discipline as other "fad" diets, but it will lose its appeal and ability to sustain if you let it get boring.

If you find yourself in a position where you have little to no info on the food you are ordering just follow the guidelines: meats, cheese, and vegetables. You can never go wrong with these keto basics and you can literally find them anywhere at any restaurant you go to.

A diet that revolves around fatty foods and still helps you lose weight is revolutionary. The more the world catches on to a healthier mind-set, we may see a rise in dining establishments providing low-carb options on their menus. So have fun with what you've learned and seize every opportunity for culinary adventure!

Keto Meal Prep

How to Save $100 and 4 Hours A Week

by Batch Cooking

Written By

Jason Michaels

Introduction

Welcome and thank you for purchasing a copy of *Keto Meal Prep.*

The world we live in today is all about hustling to the next opportunity and bustling through the inevitable daily to-do list. While we are succeeding in our careers and family life, we are failing our health by fueling our bodies with fatty convenience store snacks, and fast food eats loaded with extra sugars and carbs.

Now is not the time to blame yourself but realize that you only have one body in this lifetime and you need to begin treating it like the beautiful temple of life it is! But how does someone who is constantly busy and on-the-go eat healthier? Well, I am glad you asked!

The chapters within this book hold two incredible sources of getting your health back on track into one jam-packed book of valuable information and recipes! Let me introduce you to the ketogenic diet, paired with the awesome convenience and power of meal prepping!

The following chapters will discuss what the ketogenic diet is and how it can help you get your life back on track and feeling your best! But the best part of this book will teach you the basics of meal prepping and how it can drastically change the way you fuel your body; with meal prep, there are no excuses when it comes to choosing healthier meal choices because you already did all the work yourself!

Thanks again for your interest in how meal prepping on the ketogenic diet can change your life! Every effort was made to ensure it is full of as much useful information as possible, please enjoy!

Chapter 1: Brief Overview of the Keto Diet

This is a high-fat diet that this is low in carbs and moderate in protein consumption. The ketogenic is based on the metabolic state that you aim to get your body into, known as *ketosis*.

When your body is successfully in a ketosis state, the liver produces ketones, which become your body's main source of energy. The core of the keto is based around the idea that the human body was created to run better as a fat burner rather than a burner of sugar and carbs for energy. The ketogenic diet reverses the way in which your body functions in a positive manner. This means that it has the power to totally change your perspective on healthy nutrition!

Fat Torch Versus Sugar Burner

When you consume items that are high in carbs, such as that daily morning donut, your body has to create insulin and glucose to break it down:

- *Insulin* is created to help process the glucose in the bloodstream by transporting it throughout the body.

- *Glucose* is a molecule that is easily converted by the body as an energy source.

When glucose is the body's primary source of energy, fats are not needed, which means they are stored, also known as that pesky excess weight you want to rid yourself of. When your body uses all its glucose, your brain signals you to reach for a snack, which is typically unhealthy such as chips or candy.

This is where the ketogenic diet has the power to reverse the effects of unhealthy eating by transforming your body into a fat burner instead of a sugar burner. When you lower your consumption of carbohydrates, your body then tries to find another energy source, which is when your body enters ketosis.

When your body reaches the state of ketosis, fat cells release any water that they had been storing and the fat cells can make an entrance into the bloodstream and go to the liver. This is essentially the goal of the keto diet. Despite popular belief, you cannot enter ketosis by starving your body, but rather by not consuming carbohydrates.

Keto Diet Benefits

- More effective weight loss
- Improved cholesterol levels
- Decrease in insulin levels
- Improved blood sugar levels
- Elimination of diabetes precursors
- Decrease in the development of diseases like Parkinson's and Alzheimer's
- Treatment for cancer and growth of tumors
- Treatment for reducing symptoms of epilepsy
- Healthier skin

Foods to Avoid

- *Sugary foods*: cake, soda, candy, fruit juice, ice cream, etc.

- *Grains and starches*: anything wheat and corn-based produce such as pasta, rice, and cereals

- *Fruit*: most fruits excluding berries

- *Beans and legumes*: peas, lentils, chickpeas, kidney beans, etc.

- *Root vegetables and tubers*: carrots, parsnips, potatoes, etc.

- *Condiments*

- *Unhealthy fats*: vegetable oils, mayonnaise, etc.

- *Alcohol*

- *Anything labeled "sugar-free," "diet," or "low-carb"*: these items contain sugar alcohols that can greatly affect the success of reaching ketosis

Food to Embrace

- *Meat*: red meat, chicken, steak, turkey, sausage, ham, bacon, etc.

- *Fish*: salmon, trout, tuna, and mackerel

- *Cream and butter*: Grass-fed is the best

- *Nuts and seeds*: chia seeds, almonds, pumpkin seeds, walnuts, flaxseeds, etc.

- *Healthy oils*: extra virgin olive, coconut, avocado, etc.

- *Herbs and spices*

- *Low-carb vegetables*: green veggies, tomatoes, avocados, onions, peppers, etc.

Chapter 2: Why You Should Be Meal Prepping

There are many people that aspire to live a healthier lifestyle but have no idea where to start or have no time to spare. Eating healthy is one thing, but following through with your health and fitness goals and staying consistent is challenging.

When you have your hands full navigating life, cooking all our own meals can feel impossible, and the temptations of hitting up a fast food joint seem like an easier option.

If you are ready to reach your fitness goals, stop spending extraordinary amounts of money on junk food, then your new best friend is meal prepping!

What is Meal Prepping?

Meal prepping is planning, preparing, and packaging snacks and meals for the upcoming week with the idea of portion control and clean eating in mind. No right or wrong way happens to meal prep, which makes it a great dieting alternative for busy bees to personalize to fit into their daily schedule.

The goal of meal prepping is to save substantial time slaving away in the kitchen while having access to healthier meal options throughout the week. You simply dedicate time to planning your meals and cooking their components. Besides that, you will become *amazed* at the difference meal prepping will make in your day to day life!

Reasons Why You Should Be Meal Prepping

Effective weight loss

When you plan your meals in advance, you will know what you are putting into your body. A meal prep routine lets you control how many calories you consume, which is essential for weight loss.

Saves money

Despite popular belief, eating healthy doesn't have to be pricey. Purchasing things in bulk and taking advantage of your freezer is the key. You know exactly what to buy instead of purchasing ingredients you don't need. Plus, with meals already made, you will save a _ton_ of money on fast food meals - up to $100 a week in some cases.

Shopping is simpler

Once you plan your week's meals, grocery shopping will be a breeze since you will have a list to stick to instead of wandering around the store.

Learn portion control

Meal prep teaches you how to balance what you put inside your body. When you pack your meals in containers, it keeps you from reaching for more food that you don't need. This is essential if you want to lose weight; meal prepping allows you to control the nutrients and calories you eat.

Less waste

Meal prepping lets you utilize all your ingredients for the week before they go bad! This is a much better alternative than trashing expensive produce before you have a chance to eat it.

Saves time

While you will need to set time aside to prepare your meals, you will end up saving time in the long run. Think about it; how much time do you spend with the fridge open? How much time do you waste making a decision of what to eat just to become a victim of tempting convenience foods? With meal prep, meals are prepared ahead of time, requiring you to remove from the fridge and nuke them in the microwave. Easy!

Investment in your health

Jason Michaels *&* Thomas Hawthorn

When you can pick what you are going to stuff your face with ahead of time, you have ample time to make much healthier decisions. The benefits of eating cleaner are endless! Good nutrition is everything, especially if you are looking to fit into that bikini for the summer!

Strengthens willpower

Once you become accustomed to eating healthier, you will find that you no longer crave sugar and carbs. When you have a consistent routine of eating better, you will turn down unhealthy food choices much easier.

Reduces stress

Stress directly impacts your immune system, which can cause you to experience digestive issues, lack of quality sleep, and many more negative side effects. Coming home from work and having a meal ready to eat takes away that everyday stress!

Adds variety to your diet

Once you get the hang of meal prepping, you will feel more confident to try new recipes with new ingredients. Your taste buds will receive a variety of flavor daily.

Chapter 3: How to Avoid the 10 Most Common Meal Prep Mistakes

The way you approach meal prepping will make a world of difference when it comes to successfully implementing it into your everyday life. There are many tips out there regarding choosing recipes, shopping, and bringing it all together to create a week's worth of delicious eats.

However, you need to be aware of the things that could potentially go wrong and be knowledgeable of solutions to avoid meal prep pitfalls.

Mistake 1: Not giving yourself enough time to plan

Meal planning takes time and cannot happen in an hour. When you plan, shop, and prep as soon as you can, you are not giving yourself a sufficient amount of time to process everything, which can make it more of a stressful experience than it has to be.

- **Solution:** Allow yourself ample time to plan meals, especially as a beginner. Set aside 2 to 3 hours per week. Take advantage of the weekend to spread out planning, shopping, and prepping of meals. This will allow prepping to feel like a sustainable task that you can do for months to come. An easy way to do this at first is to make a meal calender for the upcoming week. This will help you plan efficiently and avoid wasting food.

Mistake 2: Not choosing the best recipes for your personal needs

To ensure that meal prepping works the best for you and your lifestyle, you need to understand the importance of what your body needs from the recipes you choose. If you pick a bunch of recipes that don't come close to the criteria, you will be hungry and unsatisfied.

- ***Solution:*** <u>Choose recipes</u> based on the meals you *need*. While this seems obvious, many people overlook this. Create a list of what you want recipes to do for you.

    o Need recipes to be 30 minutes or less?
    o Are you a vegetarian?
    o What ingredients do you have that need to be used?

Mistake 3: Being unrealistic and too ambitious

Meal planning should be viewed as a marathon, not a sprint to the finish. You will feel super inspired at the start of your meal prep journey, but once you start to get into the depths of planning, you can become easily overwhelmed. You need to ensure that your prep schedule matches your regular schedule so that you can sustain it.

- ***Solution:*** Begin by creating defined goals and <u>assessing your daily routine</u> and schedule; this will help you to find what is realistic for *you*. Start small and start prepping two to three nights per week. This will give you the opportunity to figure out what works and what doesn't and allows you to tweak it to your liking.

Mistake 4: Not stocking the pantry

Experienced meal planners know how essential it is to always have meal basics on hand. If you fail to keep a good supply of staple items, you will miss all the benefits of meal planning and will likely become susceptible to temptation.

- ***Solution:*** Stock your pantry with all the basics that you can use time and time again in a variety of recipes:

- o Canned goods
- o White wine vinegar
- o Pepper, salt, and other spices
- o Canned tomatoes
- o Natural sweeteners (agave, maple, and honey)
- o Coconut milk
- o Olive oil
- o Stock
- o Etc.

Even on the days, you feel like you have nothing to consume, those basic components can help you create a yummy frittata, a delicious three-ingredient entre, or a one-pot wonder.

Mistake 5: Not searching for items that need to be used up

Before you head to the store, take an inventory of ingredients you already have in your kitchen and make use of leftover components you have. It's a simple step that helps you to prevent waste and saves you money.

- **Solution:** Before choosing recipes and making a grocery list, look in your cupboards, pantry, and fridge for food that needs to be used first. Turn those greens into a tasty side before going bad or thaw that pack of chicken to create a delicious main course.

Mistake 6: Not jotting down recipes

Meal prepping is all about being organized is you want to be successful. If you fail to save or write down recipes you have enjoyed, you will fall off track and become overwhelmed.

- **Solution:** Stay organized by keeping track of recipes that you have enjoyed and new ones you want to try out. It doesn't have to be fancy; could be a scrap piece of paper or on a whiteboard in your kitchen.

Mistake 7: Not taking inventory before shopping

Once you have picked your recipes for the week, you need to see what items you already have in your pantry. This is a closely tied mistake to not seeing the ingredients that need to be used before going bad.

- **Solution:** Before heading to the store, double check your recipe and the list of ingredients. Check your kitchen to ensure you don't have any of the components already so that you prevent overbuying.

Mistake 8: Skipping pre meal prep

Pre meal prepping is obviously an essential part of meal prep; this is small tasks like organizing ingredients and labelling containers. This gives your future self a giant hand. If you skip it, you are hurting yourself and leaves more work to do on the weekends.

- **Solution:** Set aside 30 minutes to an hour of prep each evening. This will make weekend meal prep a heck of a lot more efficient.

Mistake 9: Trying new recipes each day

I highly encourage you to try new recipes, but it's also important to go about eating a new variety of foods in a strategic way. When you fill up the whole week with brand new recipes, it can become very overwhelming and hard to sustain over a long period of time.

- **Solution:** Don't throw new recipes to the side but build your meal plan around recipes you know and then add 1 or 2 new recipes per week. This will help your taste buds from becoming bored and will also strengthen your recipe collection.

Mistake 10: Failing to have a backup plan

Even the most experienced meal preppers are bound to get stuck at work or have evenings where they are not feeling like consuming the dinner they planned out. Having a plan B is essential to stay the course.

- **Solution:** Have a good backup plan and have recipes in your back pocket that you know how to make. These will be very simple and can be made quickly, such as an omelet.

Chapter 4: Delicious Keto Recipes

The following sections withhold a wide array of delicious, easy-to-make keto meal prep recipes that you will certainly want to keep in that back pocket of yours! With these recipes, you will have fewer excuses when it comes to fueling your body in a way that makes you feel better both inside and out!

Breakfast Recipes

Greek Egg Bake

Protein: 15g Fat: 11g Net Carbs: 5g Calories: 175 Fiber: 9g

Ingredients:

- ¼ cup sun-dried tomatoes

- ½ cup feta cheese

- ½ tsp. oregano

- 1 cup chopped kale

- 12 eggs

Instructions:

1. Ensure your oven is preheated to 350 degrees.

2. With the foil, line a baking sheet and with the nonstick spray, spray well.

3. Whisk the eggs and then stir in the oregano, feta cheese, tomatoes, and kale.

4. In the sheet, pour the egg mixture. Then, bake the mixture for 25 minutes.

5. Let it cool and slice.

Can be served right away or kept in the fridge for 4 to 5 days.

Turmeric Scrambled Egg Meal Prep

Protein: 29g Fat: 18g Net Carbs: 6g Calories: 216 Fiber: 11g

Ingredients:

- ½ tsp. dried parsley
- 1 cup steamed broccoli
- 2 tbsps. coconut milk
- 2 tsp. dried turmeric
- 4 eggs
- 8 pre-cooked sausages

Instructions:

1. With the nonstick spray, grease a frying pan and then place it over medium heat setting.
2. Whisk the turmeric, parsley, milk, and eggs together with a pinch of the pepper and salt.
3. In the frying pan, slowly pour the mixture of eggs. Then cook well for 2 to 3 minutes, stirring the mixture constantly to break the eggs apart.
4. Flip the eggs and cook for another couple minutes till you reach the desired texture.
5. Add the eggs to two meal prep containers and add the veggies and sausage to the containers.

Can be refrigerated for up to 5 days.

Three-Ingredient Cauliflower Hash Browns

Protein: 7g Fat: 12g Net Carbs: 3.2g Calories: 164 Fiber: 2g

Ingredients:

- ¼ tsp. cayenne pepper

- 1 egg

- ¼ tsp. garlic powder

- ¾ cup shredded cheddar cheese

- ½ tsp. salt

- 1 head of cauliflower

- 1/8 tsp. pepper

Instructions:

1. Ensure your oven is preheated to 400 degrees. Grease a tray with the nonstick spray.

2. Grate the head of the cauliflower. For 3 minutes, place in the microwave and allow to cool. Ring out excess water with the cheesecloth or paper towels.

3. Place the cauliflower with the remaining ingredients and stir well to combine.

4. On a greased tray, form the mixture into square hash browns.

5. Bake for 15 to 20 minutes.

6. Let it cool for 10 minutes.

7. Serve it warm or place into the meal prep containers.

Can be refrigerated for 4 to 5 days.

Vegan Egg Muffins

Protein: 13g Fat: 9g Net Carbs: 4.1g Calories: 143 Fiber: 6g

Ingredients:

- ¼ cup coconut milk
- ½ thinly sliced sweet onion
- ½ tsp. dried oregano or 1 tsp. fresh oregano
- ¾ cup chopped red bell peppers
- ¾ tsp. sea salt
- 1 ½ cup fresh spinach
- 8-ounce pork breakfast sausage
- 1 tbsp. extra virgin olive oil
- 9 eggs

Instructions:

1. Ensure your oven is preheated to 350 degrees. Grease a muffin tin.
2. Sauté the ground sausage, breaking up as it cooks.
3. When halfway cooked, add a tablespoon of the olive oil, along with the oregano, pepper, and onions. Sauté the mixture till the onions turn into translucent.
4. Cover the pan after adding the spinach. Cook for 30 seconds and then toss the mixture. Spinach should be wilted. Take the pan off the heat.
5. Mix the eggs in a bowl with the milk, pepper, and salt, whisking till well beaten.
6. To the eggs, add the cooked sausage and veggie mixture and mix till well combined.
7. In a muffin tin, put the mixture evenly.
8. Bake for 18 to 20 minutes.

Refrigerate for up to 4 days and frozen for up to 2 months.

Turkey Chorizo Breakfast Sandwich

Protein: 29g Fat: 11g Net Carbs: 8g Calories: 203 Fiber: 5g

Ingredients:

Turkey Chorizo:

- ¼ tsp. cayenne pepper
- 1 tsp. coriander
- ¼ tsp. dried thyme
- ¼ tsp. cinnamon
- ½ tsp. dried oregano
- ¼ tsp. pepper
- ¼ tsp. onion powder
- 1 tbsp. cumin
- 1 tsp. fennel seeds
- 1 tbsp. paprika
- 1 tsp. sea salt
- 1/8 tsp. cloves, ground
- 1-pound turkey breast, lean ground
- 1 tsp. garlic powder

Breakfast Sandwich:

- ¼ avocado
- 1 cooked turkey chorizo patty
- 1 egg
- 1 whole wheat English muffin

Instructions:

1. *To make the chorizo:* In a bowl, add the turkey and spices. Mix them well with your clean hands. Create 16 even-sized portions and make them into ¼-inch patties.
2. Cook the chorizo patties in a greased skillet till the patties turn brown.
3. *To make a sandwich:* Spray a skillet and add the egg. Cook to your preference.
4. Toast your English muffin.
5. Serve the muffin topped with one chorizo patty, eggs, and avocado.

Freeze the remaining patties to enjoy throughout the week.

Banana Strawberry Baked Oatmeal

Protein: 14g Fat: 16g Net Carbs: 7g Calories: 154 Fiber: 11g

Ingredients:

- 2 eggs
- ¼ cup pure maple syrup
- ½ tsp. salt
- 1 ½ cup chopped strawberries + more to serve
- 1 tsp. cinnamon
- 2 tsp. vanilla extract
- 3 cups almond milk
- 3 mashed/ripe bananas
- 4 cups oats, old-fashioned
- 1 tsp. baking powder

Instructions:

1. Ensure your oven is preheated to 350 degrees. Grease a baking dish.
2. Whisk the salt, baking powder, cinnamon, vanilla, maple syrup, milk, eggs, and banana together well.

3. Mix in the oats. Gently fold in the strawberries.

4. In the prepared dish, pour the mixture. Then, bake the mixture for 35-40 minutes till the oatmeal sets.

5. Before serving, allow it to sit for 5 minutes. Then, serve the topping with more chopped strawberries.

Leftovers can be refrigerated for 3 days.

Simply reheat the oatmeal with a bit of the almond milk and top with desired fruit if you so choose.

Banana Muffins

Calories: 134 Protein: 11g Net Carbs: 9.8g Fiber: 9g Fat: 4g

Ingredients:

- ¼ tsp. salt
- 1 tsp. vanilla extract
- ½ tsp. baking soda
- ½ cup unsweetened applesauce
- 1 ½ cup ripe bananas
- 3 tbsps. olive oil
- 1 tsp. baking powder
- 1 egg
- 1 1/3 cup wheat flour, whole

Instructions:

1. Ensure your oven is preheated to 375 degrees. Grease a muffin tin well.

2. Light beat the egg and then add the bananas, mashing well. Stir the remaining components, minus the flour.

3. Then add the flour, stirring gently till well combined. DON'T OVERMIX.

4. In the muffin tin, pour the batter.
5. Then, bake the batter for 22 minutes.

Muffins can either be refrigerated for 7 days or frozen for 3 months.

Vanilla Cinnamon Protein Bites

Protein: 2g Fat: 9g Net Carbs: 4.2g Calories: 112 Fiber: 3g

Ingredients:

- ¼ - 1/3 cup nut butter of choice (the creamier, the better!)
- ¼ - 1/3 cup pure maple syrup
- ¼ cup vanilla protein powder
- ½ cup almond meal
- ½ - 1 tsp. vanilla extract
- ¾ cup quick oats
- 1 tbsp. cinnamon

Instructions:

1. Grind the oats in your food processor and pour them into a mixing bowl. Add the nut butter, cinnamon, protein powder, and almond meal to the bowl, stirring well.
2. Pour in the vanilla and syrup, combining well with your clean hands.
3. With the parchment paper, like a cookie sheet, roll the mixture making 1 ½-inch balls and place on the lined sheet.
4. Freeze for 20 to 30 minutes and then place in a Ziploc baggie.
5. Dust the balls with the vanilla protein and cinnamon.

Can be refrigerated for 3 weeks or frozen for up to 6 months.

Jason Michaels & Thomas Hawthorn

Low-Carb Breakfast Pizza

Protein: 19g Fat: 16g Net Carbs: 7.2g Calories: 307 Fiber: 5g

Ingredients:

- ¼ tsp. pepper
- ½ cup heavy cream
- ½ tsp. salt
- 1 cup shredded cheese of choice
- 12 eggs
- 2 cups sliced peppers
- 8 ounces of sausage

Instructions:

1. Ensure your oven is preheated to 350 degrees.
2. Microwave the peppers for 3 minutes.
3. In a cast iron skillet, brown the sausage. Set to the side.
4. Mix the pepper, salt, cream, and eggs together and place in the skillet.
5. Cook for 5 minutes till the sides begin to become firm.
6. Place the skillet in the oven and back for 15 minutes. Then, remove the skillet from the oven.
7. To the skillet, add the cheese, peppers, and sausage and then for 3 minutes, place it under the broiler.
8. Allow to sit for 5 minutes to cool. Devour right away or split between the meal prep containers.

Can be refrigerated for 5 days or frozen for 60 days.

Blueberry Pancake Bites

Protein: 6g Fat: 13g Net Carbs: 7.5g Calories: 188 Fiber: 4g

Ingredients:

- ½ cup frozen blueberries
- 1/3 – ½ cup water
- ½ tsp. cinnamon
- 1 tsp. baking powder
- ¼ cup melted ghee
- ½ tsp. salt
- ½ cup coconut flour
- ½ tsp. vanilla extract
- 4 eggs

Instructions:

1. Ensure your oven is preheated to 325 degrees. With the butter and coconut oil spray, grease a muffin tin.
2. Mix the vanilla, sweetener, and eggs together until smooth.
3. Stir in the cinnamon, salt, baking powder, melted ghee, and coconut flour, blending till smooth.
4. To the batter, add 1/3 cup of the water and blend once more. The batter should be thick.
5. Among the muffin tin cups, divide the batter and then add a few blueberries to each muffin.
6. For 20 to 25 minutes, bake until set.
7. Allow to cool.

Can be kept in a slightly cold place in an airtight container for 8-10 days. Can be frozen for 60-80 days.

Lunch Recipes

Shredded Chicken for Meal Prep

Calories: 115 Sugar: 0g Carbs: 0g Total Fat: 4g Protein: 19g

Ingredients:

- ½ tsp. black peppercorns
- 2 bay leaves
- 2 halved cloves of garlic
- 32 ounces of chicken broth (preferably reduced-sodium)
- 4 ½ - 5 pounds skinned chicken thighs
- 4 parsley stems
- 4 thyme sprigs

Instructions:

1. Put the chicken in your slow cooker.
2. In a double-wrapped cheesecloth, place the peppercorns, garlic, bay leaves, parsley stems, and thyme sprigs. Tie off the cheesecloth and add the filled bouquet to the slow cooker.
3. Pour the broth into your slow cooker over the chicken and wrapped herbs.
4. Cover them and set to cook on low heat setting for 7 to 8 hours.
5. Discard the bouquet.
6. Place the chicken in a bowl and leave the cooking liquids in the cooker.
7. Once some of the chicken has cooled, take out the bones from the meat. Use two forks to shred the chicken, adding reserved cooking liquids while shredding to keep the meat moist.
8. Strain the remaining liquids and use for the future stock if desired.

Can be used in a large variety of meal prep recipes! To make ahead, place 2 cups of stock and chicken in separate containers.

Can be frozen for 3 months and refrigerated for 3 days.

Easy Sheet Pan Roasted Vegetables

Calories: 97 Protein: 2g Carbs: 11g Total Fat: 6g Sugar: 4g

Ingredients:

- 1 tbsp. balsamic vinegar
- ¼ tsp. pepper
- 1 chopped red onion
- 1 tsp. coarse salt
- 2 chopped red bell peppers
- 2 tsp. Italian seasoning
- 3 tbsps. olive oil, extra virgin
- 3 cups cubed butternut squash
- 4 cups broccoli florets

Instructions:

1. Ensure your oven is preheated to 425 degrees.
2. Toss the cubed squash in a tablespoon of the oil and spread out onto a baking tray. Roast for 10 minutes.
3. Toss the pepper, salt, Italian seasoning, onion, bell peppers, and broccoli till coated well.
4. Add the roasted squash to the veggies. Toss well to incorporate. Spread the veggie mixture over two baking trays.

5. Roast for 17 to 20 minutes, making sure to stir around 1-2 times throughout the cooking process. Vegetables should be tender and browned in areas.

6. Drizzle with the vinegar before eating.

Can be refrigerated for up to 7 days.

Mango Coconut Chicken Bowls

Calories: 482 Sugar: 0g Carbs: 72g Total Fat: 8g Protein: 34g

Ingredients:

- ¼ cup sweetened shredded coconut
- 1 sliced avocado
- 2 cups cooked brown rice
- 4 chicken breasts (sliced lengthwise in half)

Mango marinade:

- 1 tsp. salt
- 2 tbsps. lime juice
- 1 tbsp. Sriracha
- 2 minced garlic cloves
- 1 tbsp. honey
- 2 tbsps. olive oil
- 1 mango

Corn salsa:

- ¼ cup cilantro
- 1 can drained black beans
- ½ diced red pepper
- ¾ tsp. salt
- 1 ½ cup corn
- 1 diced red onion
- 1 tbsp. lime juice

Instructions:

1. Ensure your oven is preheated to 425 degrees.
2. Cook the rice as per the package instructions.
3. In a blender, mix all of the mango marinade ingredients together till combined.
4. Marinate the chicken in half of the mango mixture for 10 minutes.
5. Mix together the corn salsa ingredients.
6. On your baking tray, place the chicken and bake for 15-20 minutes till golden in color.
7. Slice the chicken and place into bowls, along with additional mango sauce, corn salsa, topped with the shredded coconut and cilantro. Place the avocado on top.

Can be chilled in your fridge up to 5 days.

Chicken Tikka Masala Prep Bowls

Calories: 215 Sugar: 2g Carbs: 17g Total Fat: 9g Protein: 21g

Ingredients:

- 1 ½ pounds chicken breasts (cut into 1-inch pieces; boneless, skinless)
- 1 cup brown rice
- 1 diced onion

- ¼ cup cilantro
- 1 tbsp. lemon juice
- 1 tbsp. ginger, grated
- 1/3 cup heavy cream
- 2 tbsps. tomato paste
- 1 cup chicken stock, reduced-sodium
- 2 tbsps. unsalted butter
- 2 tsp. garam masala
- 28-ounce can diced tomatoes
- 2 tsp. chili powder
- 3 minced garlic cloves
- 2 tsp. turmeric

Instructions:

1. Cook the rice in 2 cups of water following the package directions.
2. In a skillet, melt the butter. With the pepper and salt, season the chicken. Then, with the onion, add the chicken to the skillet, cooking for 4 to 5 minutes till golden.
3. Stir in the turmeric, chili powder, garam masala, ginger, and tomato paste, cooking for 1 to 2 minutes as you combine.
4. Pour the chicken stock and tomatoes in. Bring the mixture to a boil.
5. Decrease heat. Then, for 10 minutes, let it simmer, stirring on occasion.
6. Mix in the lemon juice and cream, heating through 1 minute.
7. Spoon the rice and chicken into the meal prep bowls and garnish with the cilantro.

Refrigerated for up to 7 days or frozen for 1 month.

Spinach, Tomato, and Bacon Muffin Tin Quiche

Calories: 96 Carbs: 2g Sugar: 0g Protein: 13g Total Fat: 9g

Ingredients:

- ¼ cup tomatoes, diced
- ½ cup low-fat milk
- ½ tsp. pepper
- ½ cup chopped green onions
- ½ tsp. salt
- 1 ½ cup red-skinned potatoes, diced
- 2-ounces shredded cheese of choice
- 1 ½ cup chopped spinach
- 2 tbsps. extra virgin olive oil
- 3 strips of cooked/chopped bacon
- 8 eggs

Instructions:

1. Ensure your oven is preheated to 325 degrees. Liberally grease a muffin tin.
2. Set over medium heat, warm oil in a pan. To the pan, add some salt and potatoes, stirring for 5 minutes till the potatoes are just cooked. Take it off the heat. Allow to sit and cool for 5 minutes.
3. Whisk the pepper, salt, milk, cheese, and eggs together.
4. Fold in the cooked potatoes, tomatoes, green onion, and spinach to the egg mixture.
5. Pour the egg and veggie mixture evenly in your muffin tin.
6. Bake for 25 minutes till firm to the touch.
7. For 5 minutes, allow to sit.

Can be refrigerated for 3 days and frozen up to a month.

Jason Michaels & Thomas Hawthorn

To reheat, remove the plastic wrapper, put a dampened paper towel around it, and then heat in the microwave for 30 to 60 seconds. Enjoy!

Taco Scramble

Calories: 450 Carbs: 24g Sugar: 3g Total Fat: 19g Protein: 46g

Ingredients:

- ¼ cup chopped scallions
- ¼ cup water
- ¼ tsp. adobo seasoning salt
- ½ cup Mexican shredded cheese
- ½ minced onion
- 1 pound lean ground turkey
- 2 tbsps. homemade taco seasoning (Tastier and better for you than the store-bought!)
- 2 tbsps. minced bell pepper
- 4-ounce can tomato sauce
- 8 beaten eggs

Potatoes:

- ½ tsp. garlic powder
- 1 pound red potatoes, quartered
- ¾ tsp. salt
- 4 tsp. olive oil

Homemade taco seasoning:

- 1 tsp. chili powder
- ½ tsp. oregano
- 1 tsp. paprika
- 1 tsp. cumin
- 1 tsp. garlic powder
- 1 tsp. salt

Instructions:

1. Beat the eggs, add the seasoning salt, and fold in the cheese.
2. Ensure your oven is preheated to 425 degrees. Grease a casserole dish.
3. Add the oil, salt, garlic powder, and 1-2 pinches of the pepper to the potatoes. Bake the potatoes for 45 minutes till tender, making sure to stir every 15 minutes.
4. Brown the turkey. Then add the water, tomato sauce, bell pepper, and onion. Stir, simmering for 20 minutes
5. Spray a separate skillet liberally using the cooking spray and add the eggs and ¼ teaspoon of the salt. Scramble for 2 to 3 minutes.
6. When serving, put ¾ cup of the turkey and 2/3 cup of the eggs into a meal prep container or serving bowl. Divide the potatoes among each serving with 1 tablespoon of the cheese and scallions.

Chicken Sausage and Peppers

Calories: 249 Protein: 18g Carbs: 20g Total Fat: 11g Sugar: 11g

Ingredients:

- 1 sweet onion (cut into wedges)
- 2 cups grape tomatoes
- 1 tbsp. oregano

- 1 tbsp. vinegar, balsamic
- 12-ounce package of Italian-flavored cooked chicken sausage
- 1 tbsp. olive oil
- 4 sweet peppers, color of choice (chop into 1-inch pieces)

Instructions:

1. Ensure your oven is preheated to 425 degrees. Liberally grease a baking pan.
2. In the prepared pan, add the tomatoes, onion, and peppers. Drizzle with the vinegar and olive oil and toss. Roast for 30 minutes.
3. Move the roasted veggies to one side of the tray and put the sausage in an empty portion. Roast for another 10 to 15 minutes till the sausage is heated through.
4. Sprinkle with the oregano.

Can be refrigerated for 7 days and frozen for 15 days.

Southwestern Chicken Burrito Bowls

Calories: 301 Sugar: 3g Carbs: 10g Total Fat: 14g Protein: 21g

Ingredients:

- ¼ tsp. cayenne
- ¼ tsp. pepper
- 1 ½ cup canned black beans
- ½ tsp. cumin
- ¾ cup canned corn
- 1 cup grape tomatoes
- 1 cup cooked rice
- 1 tsp. paprika

- 2 cups kale
- 3 cups shredded chicken

Instructions:

1. Prepare the rice according to the package instructions. Mix the pepper, cayenne, cumin, and paprika in with the rice when there are around 5 minutes left to cook the rice.
2. Layer your meal prep containers with the shredded chicken, rice, beans, corn, kale, and tomatoes.
3. Top with the dressing and enjoy it right away or store in the fridge for later enjoyment.

Can be refrigerated for 7-10 days.

Skinny Joes With Tangy Slaw

Calories: 381 Protein: 29g Carbs: 23g Total Fat: 14g Sugar: 4g

Ingredients:

- 1 cup chopped tomatoes
- ½ cup rolled oats
- 1 cup water
- 1 red onion, chop
- 1 green or red bell pepper, chop
- 1 ½ tsp. salt
- 1 grated carrot
- 1 tbsp. Worcestershire sauce
- 1-pound ground beef, lean
- 2 tsp. garlic powder
- 1 tbsp. olive oil

- 4 tbsps. apple cider vinegar
- 4 tbsps. tomato paste

Tangy Slaw:

- ½ chopped red onion
- ½ head cabbage
- 1 tbsp. honey
- 1 tbsp. mustard, Dijon
- 2 grated carrots
- 2 tbsps. apple cider vinegar

Instructions:

1. Press SAUTÉ. Pour the oil into an instant pot and allow to heat for a bit. Add the beef and cook till browned.
2. Push the beef to the side in the pot and add the garlic powder, salt, carrots, peppers, and onions, sautéing for 5 minutes till softened. Then pour in the water, tomato paste, chopped tomatoes, vinegar, and Worcestershire sauce. Mix well to incorporate.
3. When the mixture heats to boiling, toss in the oats. DO NOT STIR.
4. Close the lid. Press HIGH PRESSURE. For 10 minutes, cook the mixture.
5. Perform the natural release. Let it sit for a few minutes covered to allow to thicken.

1. *To make the slaw,* combine the honey, vinegar, and mustard.
2. Add the onions, carrots, and cabbage, tossing with the honey mixture.

Sloppy joe meat can be frozen for up to 3 months and refrigerated for 10 days.

Tangy slaw can be refrigerated for up to 4 days.

Mason Jar Recipes

Asian Chicken Mason Jar Salad

Calories: 524 Sugar: 15g Carbs: 39g Total Fat: 33g Protein: 28g

Ingredients:

- 1 1/3 cup halved snap peas
- 1 cup grated carrots
- 1 cup whole cashews, unsalted
- 1 julienned red pepper
- 2 cups baby spinach, sliced
- 2 cups napa cabbage, sliced
- 1 1/3 cup sliced cucumber
- 2 cups shredded rotisserie chicken
- 2 tbsps. green onions, sliced

Sesame dressing:

- 1 minced garlic clove
- 2 tbsps. rice vinegar
- 1 tbsp. minced ginger
- 1 tbsp. honey
- 1 tsp. sriracha sauce
- 1 tsp. sesame seeds
- 2 tbsps. cilantro
- 1 tbsp. olive oil
- 2 ½ tbsps. sesame oil , toasted
- 3 tbsps. low-sodium soy sauce
- *4 64-ounce mason jars*

Instructions:

1. Whisk the sesame seeds, honey, cilantro, garlic, ginger, sriracha, olive oil, toasted sesame oil, vinegar, and soy sauce together.
2. Toss the spinach and napa cabbage together.
3. Assemble the jars by adding 3 tablespoons of the dressing, 1/3 cup of the snap peas, ¼ cup of the chicken, ¼ cup of the cashews, and a sprinkle of the green onion. Serve it now or place in the fridge. *Salads last 3 to 4 days in the fridge.*

Yogurt and Granola Parfait

Calories: 98 Sugar: 4g Carbs: 2g Total Fat: 4g Protein: 5g

Ingredients:

- 2 cups granola
- 2 cups Greek yogurt (any flavor)
- 4 cups berries

Instructions:

- Layer ½ cup of the granola, ½ cup of the yogurt, and 1 cup of the berries into the jar, continuously layering till you are out of ingredients.

Can be refrigerated for 3 to 4 days.

Zucchini Lasagna

Calories: 114 Sugar: 4g Carbs: 3g Total Fat: 9g Protein: 8g

Ingredients:

- ¼ cup minced parsley
- ½ cup diced onion
- ½ pound lean ground turkey
- ½ tbsp. Italian seasoning
- ½ tbsp. minced garlic
- ½ tsp. oregano
- 1 cup part-skim mozzarella cheese
- 1 egg yolk
- 2 tsp. salt
- 1 tbsp. olive oil
- 2 zucchinis
- 6 tbsps. canned tomato sauce
- 4 tsp. parmesan cheese
- 6 tbsps. crushed tomatoes
- 8 ounces low-fat ricotta cheese

Instructions:

1. Ensure your oven is preheated to 350 degrees.
2. Slice the zucchinis 1/8-inch thick and sprinkle with 1 ½ teaspoon of the salt.
3. Bake for 15-25 minutes till the water is released from edges.
4. Lay the zucchini out on paper towels. Reduce the oven temperature to 325 degrees.
5. In a pan, warm the olive oil. Then pour turkey, garlic, and onion, cooking the meat till cooked through. Season with the seasonings. Set it aside.
6. Mix the crushed tomatoes and tomato sauce together. With the salt and pepper, season.
7. Mix the pepper, salt, egg, and ricotta together as well.

8. Layer half of the sauce between four jars. Then layer the turkey, zucchini noodles, and other ingredients. Parsley and mozzarella should go on top. Seal the jars well.

Can be refrigerated for 3 days.

Berry and Nuts Salad

Calories: 92 Sugar: 3g Carbs: 0.5g Total Fat: 7g Protein: 10g

Ingredients:

- ¼ cup chopped almonds
- ½ cup blackberries
- ½ cup blueberries
- ½ cup strawberries

Zesty Dressing:

- ¼ cup orange juice
- 1 tbsp. honey
- Juice and zest of a lemon
- 2 tbsps. olive oil

Instructions:

1. Whisk the dressing components together till blended.
2. In the mason jar, pour in 2-3 tablespoons of the dressing into the bottom. Then layer the berries, putting the almonds on the top.

Refrigerate for 3 days.

Asian Noodle Salad

Calories: 119 Sugar: 4g Carbs: 1g Total Fat: 5g Protein: 8g

Ingredients:

- ½ cup crunchy rice noodles
- 1 cup cooked/shelled edamame
- 4 green onions, sliced
- 2 carrots, peeled/shredded
- 4 ounces soba noodles

Spicy Peanut Dressing:

- ¼ cup olive oil, extra-virgin
- 4 tsp. vinegar, rice
- 2 tbsps. peanut butter
- 4 tsp. soy sauce
- 4 tsp. sambal

Instructions:

1. Whisk together all dressing components.
2. Pour the dressing into the bottom of the jar. Then layer the noodles, edamame, carrots, green onion, and noodles on top.

Refrigerate up to 4 days.

Mediterranean Salad

Calories: 201 Sugar: 2g Carbs: 2g Total Fat: 4g Protein: 13g

Ingredients:

- 1 cup whole-grain couscous, cooked
- 1 tbsp. olive oil
- 2 ounces crumbles feta cheese
- 4-5 slices artichoke hearts, marinated in olive oil
- 6-10 cherry tomatoes
- Juice of ½ a lemon
- Sea salt
- Sprinkle of dried basil, oregano, and parsley

Instructions:

1. Mix all liquid ingredients together to create a type of the dressing.
2. Pour the dressing into the bottom of the jar. Then add other ingredients to the jar as you see fit.

Refrigerate for up to 3 days.

Feta and Shrimp Cobb Salad

Calories: 192 Sugar: 5g Carbs: 2g Total Fat: 8g Protein: 11g

Ingredients:

- 1 chopped hard-boiled egg
- 1-2 handfuls baby spinach and romaine lettuce
- 1 tbsp. chopped red onion
- 2 chopped slices bacon
- 2 tbsps. avocado
- 2 tbsps. chopped cucumber
- 2 tbsps. crumbled feta cheese
- 6-8 boiled shrimps
- 8 grape tomatoes
- Vinaigrette of choice

Instructions:

1. Pour the vinaigrette into the bottom of the jar.
2. Then layer the veggies, shrimp, bacon, and cheese on top.

Refrigerate for up to 4 days.

BLT Salad

Calories: 205 Sugar: 6g Carbs: 6g Total Fat: 18g Protein: 17g

Ingredients:

- 14 croutons
- 2 cups iceberg lettuce
- 2 cups romaine lettuce
- 2 chopped scallions

- 2 chopped tomatoes
- 4 crumbled slices bacon

Instructions:

1. Whisk all dressing components together.
2. Pour the dressing into the bottom of the jar.
3. Layer the veggies, then the croutons and bacon on top and seal.

Refrigerate for 3 days.

Rainbow Salad

Calories: 109 Sugar: 0g Carbs: 1g Total Fat: 9g Protein: 15g

Ingredients:

- ½ cup raw sunflower seeds
- 1 cup sliced carrots
- 1 cup cucumber, chop
- 1 bell pepper, yellow, chop
- 1 bell pepper, red, chop
- 2 cups chopped red cabbage
- 8 cups assorted salad greens

Balsamic Dressing:

- ¼ cup chopped parsley

- ½ cup white balsamic vinegar
- 2 minced cloves garlic
- Pepper and salt
- 2 tbsps. olive oil

Instructions:

1. Whisk all of the dressing components together.
2. Drain the chickpeas.
3. Pour the dressing into the bottom of the jar. Then layer the veggies and sunflower seeds on top. Seal well.

Can be refrigerated for up to 5 days.

Spinach, Tomato, Mozzarella Salad

Calories: 184 Sugar: 3g Carbs: 3g Total Fat: 12g Protein: 11g

Ingredients:

- 10 cups baby spinach
- 10 ounces fresh mozzarella
- 1-quart grape tomatoes
- 10 tbsps. balsamic vinegar dressing

Instructions:

- Pour the dressing in the bottom of the jar.

- Load the jar with the veggies and then the cheese. Seal well.

Can be refrigerated for up to 3 days.

Dinner Recipes

Chipotle Turkey and Sweet Potato Chili

Calories: 423 Carbs: 39g Total Fat: 18g Sugar: 6g Protein: 28g

Ingredients:

- ¼ - ½ tsp. ground chipotle powder
- 1 cup diced onion
- 1 tsp. oregano, dried
- 1 sweet potato
- 1 tbsp. oil, coconut
- 1 tsp. cumin
- 1-pound ground turkey
- 2 cups chicken broth
- 2 tsp. chili powder
- 28-ounces fire-roasted tomatoes
- 3 minced garlic cloves
- Pepper and salt

Instructions:

1. Warm up the coconut oil over intermediate-extreme warmth.

2. Once the oil begins to simmer, place the turkey in a pan. Cook for 5 minutes, breaking up as it cooks.

3. Toss in the garlic and onions, cooking for 8-10 minutes till the onions turn into translucent.

4. Turn the warmth up to high. Pour in the broth, sweet potato, and tomatoes, along with the seasonings. Bring the mixture up to a boiling point.

5. Turn down the heat to a medium setting and let simmer for 10-15 minutes uncovered. The longer you allow to simmer, the bigger the flavor.

Refrigerate for 7 days and freeze for up to 6 months.

Avocado Bacon Garlic Burger

Calories: 189 Sugar: 1g Carbs: 13g Total Fat: 22g Protein: 27g

Ingredients:

- ½ tsp. pepper
- 1 cup chopped basil
- 1 tsp. salt
- 1-pound grass-fed lean ground beef
- 2 eggs
- 3 minced cloves garlic

Toppings:

- 1 avocado
- 16 pieces of bacon, cooked
- 4 slices red onion

Instructions:

1. Mix all hamburger components till well incorporated.
2. Divide the meat into four patties.
3. In a pan, warm up the olive oil.
4. Then, place the patties, grilling for 4 minutes per side.
5. Make the burgers with the avocado as the bun and other desired toppings.

Chutney Cilantro Meatballs

Calories: 375 Sugar: 3g Carbs: 23g Total Fat: 29g Protein: 35g

Ingredients:

Sauce:

- ½ cup water
- 1 chopped yellow onion
- 2 tbsps. avocado oil
- 28-ounce can crushed tomatoes

Meatballs:

- ½ cup quick-cooking brown rice
- 1 tsp. salt
- 1 tsp. ras el hanout spice blend
- 1 pound ground turkey

Chutney:

- ¼ tsp. cayenne pepper
- 1 bunch cilantro
- 1 green onion
- ¼ tsp. pepper
- 1 tsp. sesame oil, toasted
- 1 tbsp. lemon juice
- ½ tsp. salt

Instructions:

1. To create the sauce, push SAUTÉ and warm up the oil. Sauté the onion for 10 minutes. Then add the water and tomatoes, mixing well as you heat to simmer.
2. To create the meatballs, mix the salt, ra el hanout, rice, and turkey together. Form the mixture into 12 meatballs.
3. Put the meatballs in an even layer in the simmering sauce, spooning a bit of the sauce over the meatballs.
4. Place the lid on, using the PRESSURE RELEASE to seal. Press CANCEL and select POULTRY for 15 minutes.
5. While the meatballs cook, prepare the chutney by combining all chutney ingredients together, grinding them into a paste with the mortar and pestle.
6. Perform the quick release on the meatballs. Serve in the sauce and top with the chutney.

Instant Pot Lamb Shanks

Calories: 338 Sugar: 6g Carbs: 19g Total Fat: 37g Protein: 42g

Ingredients:

- ¼ cup minced Italian parsley
- 1 cup bone broth
- 1 chopped onion
- 1 tbsp. balsamic vinegar
- 1 tsp. fish sauce, red boat
- 1 pound ripe Roma tomatoes
- 1 tbsp. tomato paste
- 2 chopped celery stalks
- 2 tbsps. ghee
- 3 pounds lamb shanks
- 2 chopped carrots
- 3 smashed/peeled garlic cloves
- Pepper and salt

Instructions:

1. Season with the shanks with the pepper and salt.
2. Press SAUTÉ on the instant pot, melt a tablespoon of the ghee. Place the shanks into the pot and sear on all sides for 8-10 minutes.
3. As the lamb browns, chop up the veggies. Take out the lamb from the pot.
4. Lower the heat and add the remaining ghee. To the pot, add the onion, celery, and carrots, seasoning with the pepper and salt.
5. Add the garlic cloves and tomato paste, stirring for at least 60 seconds.
6. Place the shanks back into the pot along with the tomatoes.
7. Pour the balsamic vinegar, fish sauce, and bone broth into the pot.
8. Lock the lid. Press MANUAL and set to cook for 50 minutes. Perform the natural release.
9. Remove the shanks to the plate and top with the sauce.

Cranberry Spice Pot Roast

Calories: 312 Carbs: 13g Total Fat: 29g Sugar: 16g Protein: 54g

Ingredients:

- ¼ cup honey
- ½ cup water
- ½ cup white wine
- 1 cup frozen whole cranberries
- 1 tsp. horseradish powder
- 2 cups bone broth
- 2 peeled garlic cloves
- 2 tbsps. olive oil
- 3 to 4 pounds of beef arm roast
- 3-inch cinnamon stick
- 6 whole cloves

Instructions:

1. Dry the meat with the paper towels. Season liberally with the pepper and salt.
2. Press SAUTÉ on the instant pot. Heat up the oil and place the roast in, browning for 8-10 minutes on all sides. Remove and put to the side.
3. Pour the wine into the instant pot. Using a wooden spoon, from the bottom, scrape the bits. Cook for 4-5 minutes to deglaze.
4. Add the cloves, garlic, cinnamon stick, horseradish powder, honey, water, and cranberries to pot. Cook for 4-5 minutes till the cranberries start to burst open.
5. Place the meat back into the pot. Pour in just enough bone broth to cover the meat.
6. Lock the lid. Press HIGH PRESSURE to cook for 75 minutes.
7. Perform the natural release of the pressure for 15 minutes and then quick release the rest.
8. Place the meat on the serving platter and top with the cranberry sauce.

Jason Michaels & Thomas Hawthorn

Garlic Pork and Kale

Calories: 437 Sugar: 11g Carbs: 20g Total Fat: 31g Protein: 49g

Ingredients:

- 1 tsp. minced rosemary
- 1 tbsp. red wine vinegar
- 20-25 whole garlic cloves
- 2 sprigs of thyme
- 1 chopped yellow onion
- 2 tbsps. olive oil
- 2 ½ pound pork shoulder (boneless; cut into 1 ½-inch chunks)
- 2/3 cup red wine, dry
- 2/3 cup chicken broth

Instructions:

1. Season the pork liberally with the pepper and salt.
2. Press SAUTÉ on the instant pot and heat up the olive oil. Working in batches, sear the pork till browned. Remove with the slotted spoon. Discard the fat from the instant pot.
3. Add the thyme and onion to the instant pot, sautéing for 5 minutes. Then add the rosemary and garlic, cooking for 60 seconds.
4. Using a wooden spoon, pour wine in to deglaze the bits from the bottom of the pot.
5. Pour in the broth and add the pork back in. Combine.
6. Lock the lid. Press MANUAL to cook for around 40 minutes. Perform the quick release.
7. Stir in the kale. Press HIGH PRESSURE to cook for another 10 minutes. Perform another quick release.

8. Kale and pork should be nice and tender.

Can freeze up to 3 months.

Lemon Pepper Salmon

Calories: 174 Sugar: 1g Carbs: 29g Total Fat: 11g Sodium: 118mg Protein: 36g

Ingredients:

- ¼ tsp. salt
- ½ thinly sliced lemon
- ½ tsp. pepper
- ¾ cup water
- 1 julienned carrot
- 1 julienned red bell pepper
- 1-pound salmon filet
- 1 julienned zucchini
- 3 tsp. ghee
- Few springs of basil, tarragon, dill, and parsley

Instructions:

1. Pour the herbs and water into the instant pot. Place a trivet into the pot and gently place the salmon onto it.
2. Drizzle the fish with the ghee, pepper, and salt. Cover with slices of the lemon.
3. Lock the lid. Press STEAM to cook for 3 minutes.
4. Julienne your veggies while the salmon cooks.
5. Perform the quick release. Press CANCEL. Remove the rack with the salmon.

6. Discard the herbs. To pot, add veggies. Press SAUTÉ and cook for 1-2 minutes.

7. Serve the salmon with the veggies, along with a teaspoon of the cooking fats if you so choose.

Beef and Broccoli

Calories: 259 Sugar: 2g Carbs: 12g Total Fat: 9g Protein: 28g

Ingredients:

- ¼ tsp. fresh ginger
- 1 tbsp. cooking oil
- 10 to 12-ounce flank steak or sirloin
- 2 minced garlic cloves
- 3 ½ cups broccoli florets
- water

Marinade:

- 1 tsp. cornstarch
- ¼ tsp. dark soy sauce
- ½ tsp. sesame oil
- 1 tsp. soy sauce, low-sodium
- 1/8 tsp. pepper

Sauce:

- ¼ tsp. dark soy sauce
- ½ tsp. dry sherry
- 1 tsp. sesame oil, toasted

- 1 ½ tbsp. oyster flavored sauce
- 1 ½ tsp. soy sauce, low-sodium
- 1/3 cup water, cold
- 2 tsp. cornstarch
- 2 tsp. sugar

Instructions:

1. Mix all marinade ingredients together. Add the beef slices and let them sit for at least 10 minutes.
2. Blanch the broccoli.
3. Combine all sauce ingredients together.
4. Warm the oil in either a pan or wok. Add the beef in a single layer to sear. Pour the garlic and continue cooking the meat till cooked through. Pour the sauce in, constantly stirring till it becomes thickened. Add more water to thin it out if needed. Add the broccoli and stir everything well to coat. Season with the pepper and salt if desired.
5. Sprinkle the sesame seeds and chopped onions if desired.
6. Divide among containers.

Shrimp With Zucchini Noodles

Calories: 119 Sugar: 1g Carbs: 4g Total Fat: 8g Protein: 14g

Ingredients:

- ½ pound shrimp
- 1 tbsp. olive oil
- 4 zucchinis, spiralized

Sauce:

- ¼ cup + 2 tbsps. Thai sweet chili sauce
- ¼ cup + 2 tbsps. light mayo
- ¼ cup + 2 tbsps. plain Greek yogurt
- 1 ½ tsp. sriracha sauce
- 1 ½ tbsp. honey
- 2 tsp. lime juice

Instructions:

1. Cook the shrimp till opaque.
2. Warm up the oil in a pan and add the zucchini till tenderized. Drain and let it rest for 10 minutes.
3. Mix all sauce components together until smooth.
4. Split up the sauce into the containers. Add the zucchini noodles and gently stir to coat well. Add in the shrimp among containers.

Shrimp Taco

Calories: 215 Sugar: 1g Carbs: 3g Total Fat: 15g Protein: 12g

Ingredients:

Spicy Shrimp:

- ¼ tsp. onion powder
- ¼ tsp. salt
- ½ tsp. cumin
- ½ tsp. chili powder

- 1 tbsp. olive oil
- 1 clove garlic, minced
- 20 shrimps

For bowl assembly:

- ½ cup cheddar cheese
- 1 cup black beans
- 1 cup tomatoes
- 1 cup corn
- 1 lime
- 2 tbsps. cilantro

Instructions:

1. Mix all of the shrimp spices together. Add the shrimp, tossing gently to coat. Cover and chill for 10-15 minutes or up to 24 hours.
2. In a skillet, warm the oil and add the shrimp. Cook till cooked thoroughly.
3. To assemble the bowls amongst containers, top with five shrimps, a scoop of tomatoes, beans, corn, and a sprinkle of the cheese and cilantro and a lime wedge.

Refrigerate for up to 14 days.

Lemon Roasted Salmon With Sweet Potatoes and Broccolini

Calories: 223 Sugar: 3g Carbs: 5g Total Fat: 19g Protein: 19g

Ingredients:

- 1/8 tsp. red pepper flakes and thyme
- ¼ tsp. garlic powder
- Pepper and salt
- 2 tbsps. lemon juice
- 1 tbsp. butter
- 12 ounces of wild-caught salmon filets
- 4 cups broccoli florets
- 1-3 tbsps. olive oil
- ½ tsp. cumin
- 2 sweet potatoes, cubed

Instructions:

- Ensure the oven is preheated to 425 degrees. On a sheet pan, place the sweet potatoes on one side and the broccoli on the other. Drizzle both with the oil to the pepper, salt, and cumin and toss. Bake the potatoes for 15 minutes and put the broccoli to the side.
- Mix the pepper, salt, thyme, pepper flakes, garlic powder, lemon juice, and butter together. Heat for a few seconds in the microwave for the butter to melt.
- With the foil, line a tray, spray, and place the salmon on it. Drizzle the fish with the lemon sauce.
- Remove the potatoes, put the broccoli and salmon on the tray, and put back in the oven for another 12-15 minutes.
- Divide the veggies and fish among containers.

Dessert Recipes

Cinnamon Apples

Calories: 102 Carbs: 4g Total Fat: 3g Sodium: 24mg Sugar: 32g Protein: 13g

Ingredients:

- ½ cup brown sugar
- 1 tbsp. cinnamon
- 2 tbsps. unsalted butter
- ½ cup sugar
- 1/8 tsp. nutmeg
- 3 tbsps. cornstarch
- 6 Granny Smith apples
- Pinch of salt

Instructions:

1. Peel and thinly slice the apples.
2. Pour all ingredients into your instant pot. Stir well to combine.
3. Press MANUAL to cook for 18 minutes. Perform the natural release.
4. Stir up the mixture well and serve!

Refrigerate for 7 days or freeze for 2 months.

Stuffed Peaches

Calories: 237 Sodium: 173mg Carbs: 8g Sugar: 36g Total Fat: 11g Protein: 15g

Ingredients:

- Pinch of sea salt
- ¼ tsp. almond extract
- ½ tsp. cinnamon

- 2 tbsps. butter
- ¼ cup maple syrup
- ¼ cup cassava flour
- 5 peaches
- ½ cup slivered almonds

Instructions:

1. Cut off about ¼ inch from the top of the peaches. Remove the pits and hollow them all out.
2. Mix together the remaining components till crumbly. Pour the crumble mixture into the peaches.
3. Place a steamer basket into the instant pot. Add 2 cups of the water and place the peaches into the basket.
4. Lock the lid, press MANUAL to cook for 3 minutes. Perform the quick release.
5. Remove the peaches and allow to cool for 10 minutes.

Can be refrigerated for 4 days.

Blackberry Curd

Calories: 91 Sugar: 28g Carbs: 2g Total Fat: 0g Sodium: 11mg Protein: 1g

Ingredients:

- 2 tbsps. lemon juice
- 1 cup sugar
- 12 ounces fresh blackberries
- 2 egg yolks

- 2 tbsps. butter

Instructions:

1. Pour the lemon juice, sugar, and blackberries into an instant pot. Lock the lid. Press HIGH PRESSURE to cook for a minute.
2. For 5 minutes, perform the natural pressure release. Then quick release any remaining pressure.
3. Puree the blackberries and remove the seeds as best as you can.
4. Whisk the egg yolks and then add to the hot blackberry puree. Pour it back into the instant pot.
5. Press SAUTÉ and bring to a boil. Stir frequently. Turn off the instant pot and mix in the butter.
6. Pour into the storage container and allow to cool. Chill in the fridge until ready to eat!

Refrigerate for 7 days and freeze for up to 3 months.

Cinnamon Pecan Chia Bars

Calories: 175 Sugar: 9g Carbs: 15g Total Fat: 11g Sodium: 143mg Protein: 12g

Ingredients:

- ¼ cup almond butter
- ½ cup pecan pieces
- ¾ tsp. cinnamon
- 2 tbsps. chia seeds
- 12 Medjool dates, pitted

Instructions:

1. With the parchment paper, line a loaf pan. Allow the excess paper to hang over sides for easier removal later on.

2. In a blender, pour in all recipe components. Process till evenly distributed. The mixture should hold its shape.

3. In a loaf pan, pour mixture in. Firmly press into a block that is ½-inch thick. It will more than likely not take up the whole pan.

4. Chill for 45 minutes till the mixture has set. Slice into the bars.

Chocolate Coconut Bites

Calories: 71 Sugar: 1g Carbs: 21g Total Fat: 16g Sodium: 196mg Protein: 7g

Ingredients:

- ½ cup pecans
- 1 tbsp. cocoa powder
- ½ cup shredded coconut flakes, unsweetened
- 1 tbsp. milk, almond
- 1 tbsp. chia seeds
- 1 tbsp. collagen peptides
- 1 tbsp. liquid coconut oil
- 2 tbsps. hemp seeds
- 8 dates, pitted
- Extra coconut flakes (optional)

Instructions:

1. Blend all recipe components within a food processor till well incorporated.
2. Roll the mixture into 1-inch balls. Roll in additional coconut flakes if you so choose.

Freeze for up to 60 days.

Oatmeal Energy Bites

Calories: 71 Sugar: 1g Carbs: 21g Total Fat: 16g Sodium: 196mg Protein: 7g

Ingredients:

- ½ cup almond butter
- ¼ cup ground flax seed
- 1 cup oats, rolled
- 1/3 cup honey, raw
- ½ cup chocolate chips

Instructions:

1. Mix all recipe components together.
2. Roll out teaspoon-sized balls onto a tray lined with the parchment paper.
3. Freeze the balls for 1 hour.

Freeze for up to 1 month.

Fat Bomb Recipes

Walnut Orange Chocolate Bombs

Calories: 87 Sugar: 1g Carbs: 2g Total Fat: 9g Protein: 2g

Ingredients:

- ¼ cup extra virgin coconut oil
- ½-1 tbsp. orange peel or orange extract
- 1 ¾ cup chopped walnuts
- 1 tsp. cinnamon
- 10-15 drops stevia
- 125 g 85% cocoa dark chocolate

Instructions:

1. Melt the chocolate with your choice of method.
2. Add the cinnamon and coconut oil. Sweeten the mixture with the stevia.
3. Pour in the fresh orange peel and chop the walnuts.
4. In a muffin tin or in the candy cups, spoon in the mixture.
5. Place in the fridge for 1-3 hours until the mixture is solid.

Mini Lemon Tart Bombs

Calories: 101 Protein: 3g Carbs: 1g Total Fat: 11g

Ingredients:

Crust:

- ¾ cup grated dried coconut
- 1 ½ tsp. vanilla extract
- 1 cup almond, cashew or other nut flour
- 2 tbsps. sugar substitute
- 3 tbsps. lemon juice
- 4 ½ tbsps. melted ghee
- Pinch of salt

Filling:

- ¼ tsp. salt
- 1/3 cup lemon juice
- ½ cup softened butter or ghee
- 1 tbsp. sugar substitute
- 1/3 cup full-fat almond or coconut milk
- zest of 2 lemons
- 1 tsp. sugar-free vanilla extract
- 2 tsp. lemon extract

Instructions:

1. *For the crust:* Combine entirely crust ingredients in a medium-sized bowl together. Then roll into a log shape with the help of the waxed paper.
2. Proceed to cut into 20-24 slices.
3. Roll each slice into a ball and press gently into the tart pans.
4. Chill until you are ready to fill the crusts.

5. *For the filling:* In a food processor, pour in the butter and beat till fluffy in the texture.
6. Add the salt, zest, extracts, sweetener, lemon juice, and milk, blending until smooth.
7. Taste the mixture periodically and add more lemon juice or sweetener until it meets your taste bud needs.
8. Then pour the filling into your frozen crusts.
9. Top with a sprinkle of the lemon zest.
10. Chill until the tarts are set. Should make about 24 tarts.

Cinnamon Roll Bomb Bars

Calories: 102 Carbs: 2g Total Fat: 15g Protein: 2g

Ingredients:

- ½ cup creamed coconut
- 1/8 tsp. cinnamon

First icing:

- 1 tbsp. butter, almond
- 1 tbsp. coconut oil, extra-virgin

Second icing:

- ½ tsp. cinnamon
- 1 tbsp. coconut oil (extra virgin) or almond butter

Instructions:

1. With the liners, line a mini loaf pan or baking dish.
2. Using your clean hands, combine the cinnamon and coconut cream. Then pat into a dish.
3. In a separate bowl, mix almond butter and coconut oil together. Then spread the mixture over the creamed coconut.
4. Place in the freezer for 5-10 minutes.
5. In yet another bowl, whisk together ingredients of second icing until combined. Drizzle the icing over bars and let it freeze again for 10-20 minutes.
6. Cut into bars and enjoy!

Can be frozen for up to 3 months.

Macadamia Chocolate Fudge Bombs

Calories: 267 Protein: 3g Carbs: 3g Total Fat: 19g

Ingredients:

- ¼ cup heavy cream or coconut oil
- 2 tbsps. sweetener of choice
- 2 ounces cocoa butter
- 2 tbsps. unsweetened cocoa powder
- 4 ounces chopped macadamias

Instructions:

1. In a saucepan, melt the cocoa butter over a simmering pot of water and then add the cocoa powder. Combine.
2. Pour in the sweetener and macadamia nuts and stir well.
3. Then add the cream, mixing well and bringing the mixture back to room temperature.
4. Pour the mixture into the molds or candy cups. Allow time for the bombs to cool and chill to harden.

Peanut Butter Chocolate Bombs

Calories: 211 Protein: 3.5g Carbs: 2g Total Fat: 15g

Ingredients:

- ¼ cup chopped walnuts
- ½ cup butter or coconut oil
- ½ cup natural peanut butter, plain or chunky
- ½ tsp. vanilla extract
- 1 cup sweetener of choice
- 1/3 cup powder, cocoa
- 2 ounces cream cheese, softened
- 1/3 cup vanilla whey powder
- Dash of salt

Instructions:

1. Line a 5 x 7 dish with the parchment paper, ensuring there is an overhang of paper of two sides to aid in the removal later on. Spread the melted butter over the paper as well.
2. In a saucepan on low heat setting, melt the butter and peanut butter together, combining well.

3. In another bowl, beat the cream cheese until it soft and proceed to beat in the peanut butter until smoothened mixture.

4. Add sugar substitute and vanilla.

5. Mix together the salt, protein powder and cocoa powder in a separate bowl, sifting dry ingredients into wet ones until smooth in texture. Stir in nuts.

6. Spread the fudge mixture into the prepared pan, placing in the freezer to harden.

7. Remove and cut into squares. Store in the chilled area before serving.

Savory Mediterranean Fat Bombs

Calories: 164 Protein: 4g Carbs: 2g Total Fat: 17g

Ingredients:

- ¼ cup butter or ghee
- ¼ tsp. salt
- ½ cup full-fat cream cheese
- 2 crushed garlic cloves,
- 2-3 tbsps. freshly chopped herbs
- 4 pieces of drained sun-dried tomatoes
- 4 pitted olives
- 5 tbsps. grated parmesan cheese

Instructions:

1. In a bowl, cut butter into tiny pieces. Then add cream cheese.
2. Let it sit in room temperature for 20-30 minutes until soft.
3. Mash together with the fork until mixed. Add the tomatoes and olives.
4. Add the garlic and herbs, and season to taste with the salt and pepper.
5. Mix well ingredients together.

6. Put in the fridge for 20-30 minutes until solidified.
7. Take out the mixture and form five small balls. Then proceed to the roll balls into the grated parmesan cheese.
8. Eat right away or store in the fridge.

Bacon Guac Bombs

Calories: 156 Protein: 5g Carbs: 1g Total Fat: 15g

Ingredients:

- 4 slices of bacon
- ¼ tsp. salt
- 1 tbsp. lime fresh lime juice
- ½ small diced onion
- 1 chopped chili pepper
- 2 cloves crushed garlic
- ¼ cup butter or ghee
- ½ large avocado
- 1-2 tbsps. freshly chopped cilantro
- 1/8 tsp. cayenne pepper

Instructions:

1. Ensure the oven is preheated to 375 degrees.
2. Using the parchment paper, line a baking tray and proceed to lay out the bacon slices, ensuring none overlap.
3. Cook the bacon for 10-15 minutes or until golden brown. Remove and let it cool.

4. In a bowl, mash together the remaining ingredients together until combined. Then add diced onion.

5. Add the bacon grease and combine. Cover the mixture with the foil and put into the fridge for 20-30 minutes.

6. Crumble the bacon to use as breading.

7. Roll the avocado mixture into about six balls and roll into bacon pieces.

Salmon Bombs

Calories: 147 Protein: 3g Carbs: 0.5g Total Fat: 16g

Ingredients:

- ½ cup cream cheese, full-fat
- 1 tbsp. lemon juice, fresh
- ½ package smoked salmon or smoked mackerel
- 1/3 cup butter
- 1-2 tbsps. chopped fresh or dried dill

Instructions:

1. In a food processor, pour in salmon, butter, and cream cheese, adding the lemon juice and dill while pulsing.

2. With the parchment paper, line a tray and place the salmon mixture in 2.5 tablespoon sizes on the tray.

3. Top with the dill and put in the fridge to chill for 1-2 hours until firm.

Jalapeno and Cheese Bombs

Jason Michaels & Thomas Hawthorn

Calories: 142 Protein: 4g Carbs: 1g Total Fat: 15g

Ingredients:

- ¼ cup grated cheddar cheese
- ¼ cup unsalted butter
- 2 g halved, seeded, & chopped jalapeño peppers
- 3.5 ounces of full-fat cream cheese
- 4 slices of bacon

Instructions:

1. Ensure your oven is preheated to 325 degrees.
2. With the parchment paper, line a baking sheet, ensuring there is extra hanging over the edge to aid in removing later.
3. Mash together the cream cheese and butter in a bowl and then put in the food processor, mix until smooth in texture.
4. Lay out the bacon slices on the parchment paper, leaving a space between them. Cook for 25-30 minutes until the slices are crispy. Remove and set aside to allow to cool.
5. Add together the cheese and jalapeños to the cream cheese and butter mixture. Chill for half an hour to 1 hour until set.
6. Split up the mixture into six fat bombs and place them on the parchment paper. If serving right away, roll in the crumbled bacon. If later, chill the mixture before coating in the bacon.

Pizza Bombs

Calories: 112 Protein: 5g Carbs: 2g Total Fat: 10.5g

Ingredients:

- 14 slices of pepperoni
- 2 tbsps. freshly chopped basil
- 2 tbsps. sun-dried tomato pesto
- 4 ounces of cream cheese
- 8 pitted black olives

Instructions:

1. Chop up the olives and pepperoni.
2. In a bowl, mix all together the cream cheese, tomato pesto, and basil and add the pepperoni and olives, mixing well to combine.
3. Form the mixture into balls and then top with the pepperoni, basil, and olive.

Rice Alternatives

One of the toughest challenges when doing keto is finding substitutes for plain old white rice. Here's 10 easy ones.

Cauliflower Rice

Just mince up cauliflower to a rice-like consistency in a food processor and you're good to go. One serving even contains a day's worth of Vitamin C

Broccoli Rice

Same as above - also looks great for photos!

Green Bean Fries

Sauteed green beans with some garlic and olive oil go well with so many different meals.

Zucchini Noodles

A great way to add some more bulk to meals, ideal if you naturally need to eat a higher volume of food to stay full. Use a spiralizer to make these.

Butternut Squash Noodles

Same as above

...and the one food which isn't keto friendly - but everyone thinks is...

Quinoa!

Whether it's red, black or white quinoa, all of these have more than 30g of net carbs per serving, and as such, will usually break your state of ketosis. Avoid quinoa if you're doing keto.

Emergency Keto Meals at Popular Fast Food Chains

As much as we like to plan, it's not possible to stay consistent 100% of the time. Life gets in the way. Fortunately, most fast food chains now have keto friendly meals. Here's a few options at the big chains.

Subway

Skip the bread (duh) and opt for a salad instead. The tuna salad with cheese, black olives, green peppers, lettuce, spinach and pickles has just 330 calories and 7G net carbs. Don't bother with dressings or sauces outside of olive oil, salt and pepper - and you're good to go

Chipotle

A salad bowl with meat, tomato based salsa (no corn), sour cream and cheese is both delicious and keto-approved.

McDonald's

Pro-tip, you can order the sandwiches without bread! Some restaurants might give you a strange look. Worst case scenario you order normally and toss out the bun. The McDouble, McChicken and Grilled Chicken Sandwich are all keto friendly. As are the sausage and egg mcmuffins

Burger King

Same applies here, a Whopper or Double Cheeseburger without bread or ketchup is keto friendly.

Jason Michaels & Thomas Hawthorn

Taco Bell

This one is a little more complicated - order a side of lettuce, side of beef, side of chicken, and side or two of guacamole, then combine for a quick and cheap meal.

KFC

Protein heaven over at the colonel. Grilled chicken thighs are 17g protein with 0 carbs per piece. Breasts are 38g with no carbs. You can also get a side of green beans.

Carl's Jr.

One of the few places which actually has Lettuce-wrapped as an option. The thickburger is just 9G of carbs when you opt for this keto-friendly choice.

Jimmy John's

Any of their sandwiches can be made as Unwiches (order a slim one if you want a save a few bucks) which means no bread.

Five Guys

Same as Carl's Jr. Just order the lettuce wrap options and you're good to go.

In-n-Out

Order your burger "protein style" - a hamburger, cheeseburger or double double comes it at 11G of net carbs with this method.

Chapter 5: Methods to Properly Store Food

Congratulations! So far you know the ins and outs of the ketogenic diet, meal prep mistakes to avoid, and a nice array of keto meal prep recipes to get you started! Now, it's time to discover the proper way to store your deliciously prepped meals so that you can enjoy them as if they were fresh off the press!

Pantry Tips

There are many other items besides fruits, veggies, and canned goods that can reside happily in a pantry. These tips pertain to the foods in storage that don't need to be frozen or refrigerated:

- To lengthen the time of prepper foods, store them in the plastic or glass meal prep containers

- Most canned foods that are low in acid, such as vegetables, crab meat, and tuna can last up to 2 to 5 years. Ensure you check the date.

- Canned foods that are high in acid, like the tomato-based items, pineapple, and grapefruit have a shelf life of 12 to 18 months.

- Conditions of storage areas should be cool, dark, and dry with temperatures that range from 50 to 70 degrees. Warm climate makes the food deteriorate faster, so keep the items away from the hot pipes, dishwasher, and oven.

Fridge Tips

- Stay alert for spoiled food. If anything looks or smells off, it should be thrown out. Yes, mold can happen in the fridge too.

- Keep the prepped meals covered and in the plastic or glass containers, wrapped in the foil or plastic wrap.

- Pay attention to the expiration dates.

- Be vigilant of the 2-hour rule of refrigeration, meaning not leaving items that require to be chilled out for more than 2 hours, such as dairy, seafood, eggs, meat, chicken, etc.

- Set the temperature in your fridge to 40 degrees or lower.

Freezer Tips

I want to nicely remind you that freezing meals does not kill bacteria, but it can stop it from growing. Most frozen foods can last for a long time, but the color, flavor, and tenderness of the frozen items can be affected the longer they are frozen.

- Thaw food in your fridge before prepping

- Don't fear the freezer burn; it's a quality of food issue, not a food safety problem

- Label all packages you freeze with the date, what food is in it, and any other identifying information that will help your meal prep efforts, such as what it weighs or how many servings are in the container
- Ensure that you properly wrap the food you wish to freeze, utilize the airtight storage containers, and use the bags, plastic wrap, and foil that is freezer-grade
- Set the temperature of your freezer to 0 degrees or below

Freezer vs. Fridge

Not all edibles are freezer friendly:

- Fruits high in water content
- Lettuce
- Uncooked batters
- Eggs
- Cooked pasta
- Soft cheeses
- Cultured dairy

Freeze your meals if you don't plan to consume them in 3 to 4 days after you prepare them. Remember that the prepping frozen meals take a bit more preparation time than refrigerated meals.

- Thaw out meals for a few hours or overnight before heating and consuming

- Frozen meals last substantially longer than refrigerated meals, some being able to be frozen up to 1 year

Refrigerated meals are capable of being tasty, fresh, and convenient for a few days. After prepping, you just have to nuke the meals in the microwave. After several days of living in the fridge, however, meals can lose their freshness, taste, and moisture. This is because dry air circulating takes the moisture out of the food.

Refrigerate the meals you plan to eat in 3 to 4 days.

Chapter 6: Meal Prep Kitchen Essentials

Setting the time aside each week to prep meals for the entire week is a great way to eliminate the cravings for unhealthy eats and keep you on the right track to achieving your health and fitness goals.

Many people avoid the task of meal planning and prepping simply because they think of it as another chore; this is because they are using the wrong kitchen tools to get this big job done. This chapter will share the essential tools you need to simplify the process of meal prepping and make it more manageable.

High-quality knives

One of the most crucial tools to meal prep is having a decent set of knives that allow you to slice, dice, chop, and chiffonade like a master chef! If you have dull knives in your kitchen drawers, you are *asking* for prepping disaster. Sharp knives will save you time and make meal prep a lot easier on your hands. I recommend stainless steel knives for longevity!

Measuring spoons and cups

If you are meal prepping around macro measurements, it's very crucial to ensure you are measuring correctly. Measuring cups can help you measure dry ingredients like nuts and seeds while measuring spoons will help measure spices.

Food scale

Jason Michaels *&* Thomas Hawthorn

Even though the majority of people can easily get away with measuring with cups and spoons, there are some people that need to ensure accuracy with a food scale. These are also helpful to measure proteins.

Good kitchen utensils

Having good quality kitchen utensils is obviously essential for breezing through meal prep! When you have well-rounded utensils, you can better prepare a variety of meals with ease.

Cutting boards

Almost all meal prep recipes involve dicing, cutting, or chopping, so you need one of these at arm's length always.

Mixing bowls

Good mixing bowls are used to mix batters, marinate proteins, and much more.

Colander

Good for draining veggies and aiming for clean-tasting produce. You want crispy, rainbow-like vegetables, right?

Grater

Meal preppers love graters! It allows them to add lots of flavors to any recipe with a few simple swipes. Zest a lemon, shave some chocolate, grate a bit of nutmeg, etc.

Baking dishes

- Round cake pans
- 13 x 9 baking sheet
- 8 x 8 and 9 x 5 loaf pans
- Muffin pans
- Etc.

Non-stick skillet

Skillets are highly versatile, and you can cook just about anything in them with a little bit of fat.

Cast iron skillet

An amazing gadget for the keto diet, this skillet is capable of adding flavor and iron to your meals.

Sauté pans

Saucepan with lid

Sheet pans

Roasting pan

Cook an amazing evening meal that makes a ton of leftovers! You can even make extremely large batches of items such as granola.

Cooling rack

Spiralizer

Obviously regular pasta is not keto friendly, but a better, healthier alternative can be created with the help of spiralizing vegetables like zucchini. Yum!

Food Processor

Don't want to chop your veggies? Stick them in a food processor! Great for making pesto, hummus, dips, shredding chicken, etc.

Crockpot

Crock pots are a meal prepper's *dream* appliance; if you want to further your meal prep skills, you can save even *more* time with these babies and can make a large variety of meals and desserts.

High-speed blender

No matter if you are making the nut butter, sauces, soups, or smoothies, a good blender is a must and can help you blend in seconds!

Meal prep containers

Quality meal prep containers are an essential staple to the meal planning world. You want ones that are durable and that you can use consistently for a long period of time. Opt for containers with lockable lids rather than the standard lids which can fall off because of condensation.